MW01144204

SOS Sun

Source for Vitamin D, Happiness, Health, Wealth, Light, Weather and Climate

Big Business Based on Fear
Sun Protection, Cancer and Climate Change

Elisabeth J. Ellmer

DEDICATION

To the most powerful sources

"LOVE and LIGHT"

Elisabeth J. Ellmer

Sun Energetics mc^2

Quality of Life from the Source

www.sunenergetics.com

CONTENTS

ACKNOWLEDGMENTS

A special thanks from the bottom of my heart to everyone I met on my path of life and to all those who have contributed therefore to my development. This book could have never been accomplished without them. Every encounter, no matter how insignificant or small, whether positive, negative, critical or harmonic has made its contribution to my quest of challenging life and our reality.

Thanks to my family for their sedulous patience and support in the regards of scientific, professional and emotional areas.

Thanks to all of my readers for their interest in the topic, may it lead on to further discussions!

We all have the power to perceive our life in a different light as soon as we accept that challenge and remember our roots.

Sincere thanks to all, who contributed to this book,
Sunny regards
Your Author
Elisabeth J. Ellmer

www.jutta-ellmer.com

www.sunenergetics.com

PREFACE

"Human intelligence has grown accustomed to weak candlelight and can no longer bear to look into the sun's light."
Khalil Gibran – Philosopher – 6.1.1883 (Becharré in the Libanon) – 10.4.1931 (New York)

You are holding the right book in your hands if your personal energy levels are low and your electricity bill is too high.

With my following text and research I would like to give you the opportunity to check your behavior patterns concerning the natural association with the sun and therefore our light and energy source which subsequently lead to health. The text contains facts which are barely communicated, some are even partly and intentionally kept from the public. These facts, however, are very important for leading a balanced life, your finances and our entire future. Many parts of this information are required in order to be able to arrive at an autonomous, open-minded opinion concerning the sun. I would like to assist you in taking the most reasonable decision for long lasting health. Therefore, you need more information than what is provided by our governments and the media. The way in which you handle the text, the sun, our energy technologies, the alleged climate change and your health, as well as, the future of humanity is in your hands.

Elisabeth J. Ellmer

INTRODUCTION

There would be no life on planet Earth without our sun. However, the modern human has marked it as its enemy. The fears of UV-rays and risks involved in developing skin cancer, as well as, the alleged change in our climate has been discussed time and again so we have started to forget the importance the sun plays in our lives; meaning a healthy and fulfilled life.

During the last decades people's habits have changed dramatically around the globe. A steadily increasing number of us live in metropolises where we hardly get to see the sun. We live with fluorescent light-bulbs, which are prescribed by our governments, and work in artificial light conditions. We eat synthetically grown food, change our bio-rhythm according to the regulations of public laws, and wonder about the ever increasing cases of illness.

If the human species does not want to fade, it is time to show our colors. We should utilize the strengths of our sun to charge our energy levels and we should start to enjoy sunrises and sunsets again. The regular exposure to the sun improves one´s well-being and moods.

Yet, the discussion regarding our alleged change in climate also needs some sunny, enlightened and honest arguments coupled with a well-founded and affordable energy supply.

This book provides you with essential clues concerning the exposure to our sun, our light and energy sources. It presents enlightening information which is of great importance to each and every one of us leading to a healthy, balanced and affordable life.

Elisabeth J. Ellmer

1. No Life without the Sun

Myths, Legend and Science

The modern society has adopted a relatively negative position towards our sun compared to ancient cultures. Yet life on our planet Earth would not be possible without the sun. The energy of the sun allows plants to exist. They produce our oxygen and serve us and animals as a source of food. Furthermore, the plants provide us with fuel and building materials like timber and fossil fuels such as coal, mineral oil and natural gas.

In addition, the sun steadily dispenses us with light and warmth, and has done so for millions of years. Only minor variations in solar radiation have the power to trigger a new ice age. The variations that can be measured today are at approximately 0.1 percent. Further variations are caused by the solar cycle, which has been known to take several longer lasting breaks during the past centuries. For example, during the time period of 1650 and 1710 the sun was less powerful than usual. During that time Germany experienced long and very cold winters. However, the time period between 1100 and 1250 was very different. The sun was very active, and winegrowing was possible in Norway, and Greenland was green. You will find further information on this topic in the chapter on climate change. Only 0.1 percent of the sun's energy suffices to produce 200 billion tons of plant life. The fruits and vegetables which we consume we dedicate to the sun just as well as our flowers, trees and seaweeds. They all contain a part of the precious sun´s energy, which is so desperately required for us to lead a healthy life.

Our ancestors, who did not have the technical and scientific resources of our modern times, which has led to the current state of exciting research and new scientific findings, worshiped our sun with fervor. They purely intuitively sensed the huge impact of the sun on all forms of life. The sun was worshiped by humans as a god and very soon it´s regularity was discovered. People used the know-how of the daily recurrence as well as the annual rhythm to develop the very first calendars.

One of the most impressive buildings being linked to that is

Stonehenge in England, which was built approximately 2000 years before Christ. Blocks weighing 48 tons and measuring eight meters in height were transported over a distance of 225 kilometers in order to build this, by today's perspective, brilliant Stone Age computer. The heavy blocks are arranged in a circle that is exactly positioned for matching our seasons.

The Heel-stone and the Trilithons in Stonehenge are aligned to meet the positions of the solstice and the day and night equinox. For this reason it is believed that Stonehenge represents an observatory from ancient times. The alignment was carried out in such a way that on the morning of

Midsummer Day, when the sun reaches the most northern position during the course of the year, the sun will rise directly over the Heel-stone and the sunrays will penetrate into the inside of the building. It is highly unlikely for this precise alignment to be a coincidence. The most northern rising position of the sun is in direct dependence to the geographical latitude. In order to achieve such a precise alignment the geographical latitude of 51° 11′ had to be very well calculated or it had to be determined through observation.[1] It is very accurate and precise architecture and it would be difficult to reconstruct it with modern technologies.

The famous author and scientist of paranormal phenomena Erich von Däniken firmly believes that such a masterpiece must have been constructed by extraterrestrials. Furthermore, he discovered highly developed astronomical findings in the early civilizations of Middle and South America. These state that the mechanism of the so called "Mayan Calendar" came into being on August 11, 3114 BC, and it is believed to be more accurate than our present calendars. The author constructed a model system consisting of wheels in order to comprehend the functions of the calendar. According to that, it ends in the year 2012. Erich von Däniken assumes that the extraterrestrial builders will then return. However, the curious question of whether our contemporary calendar is correct and whether it really correlates with the "Mayan Calendar" remains.

Human kind has been studying the sun for millenniums. The oldest sun-observatory is estimated to be 7,000 years old. It can be found in Goseck, Saxony-Anhalt, Germany.

In ancient Egypt the sun god Rea was honored. The Pharaoh Ikhnaton nominated the solar disc as a divinity at about 1300 BC.

The Incas in the Andes of South America admired the sun and dedicated temples to it. The ancient Greeks called their god Helios. On a daily basis, he crossed the skies in a beautiful sun-carriage drawn by graceful horses. In astrology of the antiquities the sun stood as a symbol of vitality. The sun's positive power was repeatedly reported in the ancient world. The Assyrians already enjoyed a sun bath and the Romans reveled in an advanced bathing culture.

In China the sun was perceived as a symbol of the East, spring, masculinity and the birth of an emperor. The Germanic tribes worshiped the sun goddess "Sunna". Sunna is the personification of the sun, which provides us with light and warmth (Sol, Soll, north."Sonne"). Sunna's symbol is the sun wheel. A belt buckle showing the symbol of the sun wheel was found in Northern Germany, in the Thorsberger Moor. Experts believe the artifact can be dated to a period between 100 to 400 BC.

2

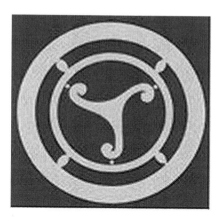

The Celts called their sun goddess Sulis, in Norway she was named Sol and the British honored the sun on Silbury Hill, the famous artificial mountain in the region of the giant Huns-graves of Avebury.

The sun was intensively honored in many cultures, as it is still today. Likewise, the Native Americans in the prairie. Every year they perform a four day sun dance called "Lakota-Sundance." Young men are accepted as fully fledged tribe members after completing the dance. Others pray for revelation regarding their life-vision and others still pray for pain relief.

The Australian Aboriginal people have a very different approach. The mother sun exists in their culture as a creation myth. In the myth, the beautiful mother sun slept for a long time below ground before being gently awoken by the Lord-father. Subsequently, the sun created all life on Earth. It presents all creatures on Earth with sufficient hours of light, during which they can arrange their affairs, and a time of darkness in which to relax from all the endeavors of the bright day.

In southern Africa the white lions were presumed to be the symbol of the sun. The tribal chiefs attributed the sun-animals with high powers and worshipped them as divine creatures with transcendent strength. Unfortunately, many of the "Sun-Lions" have been killed by poachers because of their beauty and rareness. The last specimens went extinct in the wild in the 1970s! Today, they can be found in national parks like the Kruger National Park in South Africa.

Further legends can be found in Europe. One of the prettiest festivals, is the solstice celebration in winter, which announces the change in season. From this moment on the days become longer again and the sun gains in strength.

During the solstice celebration in the summer the traditional alpenglow is held. At night flambeaus are erected on the mountain tops of the Alps to be dedicated to the sun. It is a spectacular event in upper Bavarian culture. From this moment on the days become shorter again and the sun loses in strength.

Many rituals from ancient times are still present in our day, although, first signs of physical explanations appeared as early as ancient Greece. Probably the oldest assumption originated from Xenophanes, who called the sun a fiery mist or cloud. That expression was highly risky because the ideology of the time was a contrasting one. For the first time the sun had been perceived as an object and not as a god. Other philosophers soon followed Xenophanes' opinion. Anaxagoras described the sun as a glowing rock.

The ancient Greeks already believed the Earth rotated around the sun. However, that knowledge was deliberately destroyed by the "One-God-Religion" of the Vatican as well as Allah's "One-God-Religion". Therefore, the ancient view of the world believed the planet Earth had to be the center of the Universe. The sun, the moon and planets rotate in exact orbits around the Earth. These old patterns of belief were upheld in Europe for almost 2000 years. The church defended that world view for a very long time because, due to the Bible, it is the sun which moves.

Nikolaus Kopernikus (1473 – 1543) used a mathematical model to explain the sun was at the center and the planets rotate around it. That encouraged further studies which the church disapproved of. However, due to the introduction of telescopes and the discovery of the laws of the celestial mechanics, the new view of our world came to be accepted slowly. Today we know the sun is the only star in our solar system and everything rotates around it. The sun's planets circle in orbits around the very heavy sun. Due to the sun being the fixed point in our solar system and the Earth rotating around the sun (the axis of the Earth is tilted by 23.5° to the rotation level around the sun) our seasons occur. And since the Earth is rotating around its own axis, day and night occurs.

Over 99 percent of the total mass of the solar system is attributed to the sun itself. The sun is 109 times larger than the Earth and it is believed to be 1.4 million kilometers in diameter. Despite being in a distance of 150 million kilometers from the Earth, the sun can give us light and warmth. It consists of a cocktail of light gases which are constantly on the move. The largest part, approximately 70 percent, consists of hydrogen and about 28 percent helium.

The difference is made up of a composition of various metals. It is all in constant flux and the sun transforms hydrogen nuclei into helium nuclei. During that process energy is set free which is transported from the solar core towards the surface, and from there it is radiated into outer space. These are the rays that reach the Earth.

Today, it is believed that the sun is 4.6 billion years old and that it was created due to a gravitational collapse of an interstellar gas cloud. Based on nuclear, and astrophysical laws, it is assumed the sun might become 12.5 billion years of age.

The observations concerning solar energy were first described about 75 years ago. Ernest Rutherford interpreted the correlation between radioactivity and nuclear transformation. Arthur Stanley Eddington concluded the inside of the stars´ elements melt and mix and therefore form new ones. During this process energy is released. Spectroscopic analyses have mainly found hydrogen. Only in the year

1938 Hans Bethe managed to describe the proton-proton-reactions which take place in the inside the sun. After all, we can see how young all of those scientific findings around the sun's myth really are. It is possible our modern method of approach will still be revolutionized!

Well, let us stick to what we already know. We know that day and night, as well as, the change in seasons are bound to the Earth's rotation around its own axis and the sun. It is the radiation angle with the sun which determines whether we experience spring, summer, autumn or winter. Here you can already see the enormous impact the sun has on our entire Earths climate, our weather, life, bio-rhythm and well-being. The following chapters will give you a more detailed insight into these circumstances.

On February 11, 2010, NASA launched a new solar observatory into space from its headquarters in Cape Canaveral Florida.

Until today the sun has been an unpredictable and unsettled orb offering many turbulences and surprises for science. The solar dynamic observatory (SDO) ought to improve our renewed awareness toward the sun. The data obtained from the probe will assist the prognoses of solar weather forecasts. Furthermore, answers are expected concerning the eruptions on the surface of the sun which influence our technologies as well as our satellites and our electric power supply.

For many years China has been researching various space projects as well. The sun has been observed and diagnosed by three space crafts since 2012. In this process, the interaction between the sun and the Earth is being explored. China planned the year 2012 a long time ago because the solar activity has been said to be at its next maximum at that time.

Taking a closer look at the age of the sun and the research done by human kind it becomes very obvious there is still a lot to be discovered and understood.

Despite the knowledge concerning the sun's importance for us and our planets lifespan, we have declared it to be an enemy for mankind during the past decades. Where do such accusations come from and what is the hidden agenda? Do we have to change our orientation rapidly? Read on!

2. The Concept of the Enemy Sun

Ozone Depletion, Ultraviolet Rays, Skin Cancer, Sunscreens

Solar activity, climate change, ultraviolet rays and skin cancer are keywords of our current Zeitgeist. Despite the knowledge that we owe our existence to the sun, we criticize it in many ways and mark it as hostile to man. In 2010, the Federal Institute for Health and Safety of the Federal Republic of Germany published a case study which concluded that frequent work outdoors increases the risk of skin cancer. The self-protection mechanism of our skin is so small employers were asked to take responsibility for their staff members.[3]

Furthermore, we will find many info portals on the internet from the pharmaceutical industry. All warnings on their research sound, more or less equally dramatic. We should wear protective, tightly woven textiles, long sleeved tops and long trousers. Sunglasses and hats should never go amiss. If we expose ourselves to the sun for too long it might lead to sun burn, sun allergies, light sensitivity reactions, early aging of our skin, eye diseases like eye cataracts and snow blindness.

You should plan your outdoor activities carefully and you should avoid sun radiation between 10 am and 4 pm. Sunscreen products should be used on a daily basis in order to protect us from the sun and not to forget the skin cancer screening, which are available free of charge for all men and women with state insurance coverage from the age of 35 in Germany.

We are continuously being warned about the dangerous UV rays due to ozone depletion. If one has an infectious disease, UV-B radiation will set to weaken the immune system and therefore our body´s resistance. Due to the decreasing ozone layer during the past years the UV-B rays have increased on Earth. A report from the Bavarian State Office for Environment from 2002 states that the total ozone layer above Germany has decreased by 10% since 1968 and therefore the UV-radiation increased by 15%.[4]

The Australian Government confirms that the country has the highest skin cancer ratio in the world. Over 1,700 Australians die every year due to skin cancer and two out of three Australians will develop skin cancer before the age of 70.[5]

However, even a less at risk country like Germany is highly concerned about the rapidly increasing figures of skin cancer. Generally, science distinguishes between black skin cancer (maligns melanoma) and white or non-melanoma skin cancer (basal cell carcinoma and squamous cell carcinoma).

The World Health Organization (WHO) estimates that annually two to three million new cases of non-melanoma skin cancer will be reported and 130,000 new cases of black skin cancer. As mentioned before, the highest ratio of increase is measured in Australia with an annual value of 50 to 60 new cases per 100,000 residents. In the USA about 10 to 25 people per 100,000 residents will fall ill and in middle Europe about 10 to 12 people per 100,000 residents. In Germany about 15,800 people will suffer annually from black skin cancer resulting in one percent of all deaths caused by cancer. The non-melanoma skin cancer is not fully documented in Germany. However, epidemiological studies show about 120 people out of 100,000 residents fall ill annually. Out of those, about 100 cases are related to the basal cell carcinoma, which is one of the most dangerous tumors for humans.[6]

It is important for us to know that all types of skin cancer can be treated successfully if diagnosed in time. The human skin reacts very sensitively to UV-B radiation, which very quickly causes a sun burn. Not only is our skin UV-sensitive, but also our DNA and our genetic make-up, though only in conjunction with the shorter wavelengths. Let us take a closer look at the ultraviolet radiation. Science distinguishes between three groups of ultraviolet radiation, UV-A, UV-B, UV-C. The first group of UV-A rays is measured at a wavelength of 315-400nm. These rays can penetrate right down to a human's dermis. They will not cause any inflammation or pigmentation on the skin.

The shorter and energy richer UV-B rays (315-280nm) are the ones, which are dangerous to our skin. They manage to penetrate right down to the epidermis and can therefore cause damage to the cells. The even more energy rich UV-C rays (100-280nm) are not found within the sunlight's spectrum of the Earth's surface as they are usually blocked by the ozone. However, they do occur in artificial light, as well as in the process of welding. UV-C can highly irritate the conjunctiva and it is therefore necessary to wear protective glasses.

The importance of our sun in respect to our health, well-being and survival will be revealed within the following chapters. Without getting ahead of myself, I would like to ask you to take a very critical standpoint in view of all this scare mongering be banded around.

We should ask ourselves some very simple questions. If Australia is the most effected country in regards to skin cancer and the sun is so dangerous, how did the Aboriginal people manage to live on and around that continent for more than 60,000 years and in fact without any sun cream, long-sleeved garments and all the other afore mentioned protection scenarios? They did not develop skin cancer, allergies and eye diseases. The same question applies to all Europeans whose ancestors worked under clear skies for 80 percent of their time. How could they survive so much sun? The answers are disclosed within the following chapters. However, let us start with the most simplistic one. Our skin has developed corresponding protection mechanisms against such factors. These are the swelling of the horny layer and the pigmentation by melanin (we tan). However, the protective functions are dependent on our type of skin. We distinguish between four skin types:

Skin type A) very fair skin, often with freckles, blue eyes, red-blond hair. This type runs a very high risk of getting sunburned, often after just a few minutes during the summer season.

Skin type B) fair skin, often blonde hair and grey-blue or green eyes. That particular type runs a risk of developing a sunburn after only 10 to 20 minutes of sun exposure during summer.

Skin type C) brownish skin, dark blonde or brown hair, grey or brown eyes. Sunburn will most likely only develop after 20 to 30 minutes of sun exposure during summer. That particular type can usually expect to achieve a very even tint.

Skin type D) brownish skin, mostly dark or brown hair and eyes. This type will very rarely develop sunburn and should be able to stay in the sun for up to 40 minutes without protection during the summer. The skin will brown very quickly.

For how long we expose ourselves to the sun is dependent on our skin type and is our own responsibility. Our skin certainly has the natural functions to adapt to our environment.

Yet, what has changed in modern time that make those natural mechanisms seem to be insufficient? First, our lifestyle nowadays takes place indoors for 80 percent of the times because of modern working facilities, within office blocks, factories etc. Shiftwork is taken for granted.

At an early age, our children visit crèches, kindergarten followed by schools and universities. In times gone by, scholars used the holidays to assist on the farms; today many of them spend their spare time in cinemas and with computer games. The older generation very often spends their sunset years in retirement villages and rest homes where sun light is in short supply.

Since the 20th century, we have added additional sources to the ultraviolet radiation of our sunlight, namely the artificial ones.

We all know them: the solariums with predominately UV-A radiation. In order to be able to tan that way we have to expose ourselves to higher radiation scales and thus the very sensitive cycle will come full circle. This has resulted in a solarium ban for children and teenagers under the age of 18 in Germany. The latter has been published in the official gazette of the Federal Republic of Germany on August 3, 2009. A ruling from the International Agent for Cancer Research (IARC) backs this new law, an organization within the World Health Organization (WHO), which has categorized natural and artificial UV-radiation as the highest risk factors for cancer.[7]

Long-term skin damage often only becomes apparent after 20 to 30 years. In other words, – the damage which is reported in today's statistics, might already have had their roots in the 70´s or 80´s. Artificial UV radiation is not only used in solariums. Medical science likes to utilize the inactivation effect of bacteria and viruses via UV radiators. Additionally, the newly legislated lighting, the energy saving halogen lights, has a much higher UV-radiation compared to their predecessors, the harmless light bulbs. That is why the Authorities for Radiation Protection recommend consumers to maintain a distance of at least 30 cm to the new lighting source. However, this is a little tricky when it comes to desk lights and reading lights. You will find a detailed elaboration in the chapter about the sunlight and artificial lighting.

Research done on ultraviolet rays published in the Science Daily on June 4, 2010 brought new evidence to light. Research conducted under the supervision of Eric Wolf at the University of Colorado, Boulder USA shows the early Earth was immersed in some sort of an atmosphere, which protected the surface, and therefore all life from the very dangerous ultraviolet rays for a short time after its formation about 4.5 billion years ago. A similar ultraviolet shield surrounds the Saturn moon Titan. That way, Titan is protected in the same manner from our sun's ultraviolet rays.[8] Nowadays, we talk about the ozone layer without this life onshore would not be possible for man or beast. This layer has the characteristic to absorb the dangerous ultraviolet radiation of our sun. Chemical reactions have been taking place within our atmosphere since the beginning of our planet Earth. Everything interacts and we still know only very little about long term processes. Until today, we are reliant on model calculations and there are no long-term studies available in order to combine possible causes and effects to make reliable forecasts. However, what we do know with certainty is that there are ozone holes mainly above the Antarctic, which may result in harmful ultraviolet radiation from our sun hitting the surface of earth. It is this radiation, which is being blamed for the increased incidents of skin cancer.

The exclusive responsibility for changes in our atmosphere is squarely laid at our feet, people like you and me. Humans discharge gases into the atmosphere, which have an impact on the ozone layer and therefore our lives. Chlorofluorocarbons (CFC) play a radical role in this process. In the past, these gases have been used particularly as a blowing agent in spray cans or a cooling fluid and for the production of foam materials. The usage of such substances has been widely condemned.

Unfortunately, the ordinary citizen is hastily thrown under the bus, whilst people in power remain silent behind drawn curtains. It is little known to the public for example that solid-fueled rockets are releasing huge amounts of hydrochloric acid within their emissions cocktail. The most famous rocket is the "Space Shuttle" from the 80s. Each Shuttle flight produces 187 tons of ozone damaging chlorine-gas, 7 tons of nitrogen, which also depletes the ozone layer and 387 tons of carbon dioxide (CO_2). During the 1980s, about 500 to 600 rocket launches on average per year took place globally. In 1989, before the Second Gulf War, 1,500 launches were registered.[9] The Soviet aviation engineer Walerij Bfudakow calculated the Space Shuttle launches have had a significant impact on the ozone layer.[10] If we now add the multiple nuclear tests and the abuse of our atmosphere through dangerous experiments as well as, our current topic "climate – engineering" we should arrive at a more realistic picture concerning the impacts on our environment and therefore all our lives. More information will follow in the chapter on sun activity and climate change.

With so much fear mongering in place it is time to take a good look at the alleged range of unavoidable sun protection.

3. How much Sun Protection do we really need?

Should we protect ourselves from the protection?

Wow, what an unrestrained campaign against the formerly most natural, pristine and vital object namely our sun. Do we not owe our existence to the sun? Was there not a time during which humankind lived as hunters and gatherers, eking out an existence from agricultural and stock farming and therefore with the sun? Think about ancient Rome, where sunbathing and wearing loose garments was part of the culture!

If there is just a little truth within the history of evolution, should humans and the sun not form a perfectly synchronized team? Is it not rather true that we the people of the industrial nations do not get enough sun?

Migration into cities seems an inexorable task. Ever-increasing amounts of people live and work in cities between concrete skyscrapers with only little sun available. Living space becomes increasingly smaller and we very often find the only affordable residential properties on the shadowy sides, without balconies. Even the shopping takes place in huge shopping complexes with artificial lighting, and the journey to work, kindergarten or school is taking place in cars, tubes etc. We barely walk or use our bikes. When are we going to meet this so essential sun? Maybe you had the opportunity to stay in Singapore for a little while. There, it is possible to stroll underground for hours on end from one shopping mall to another. While shopping, one often forgets whether it is morning, noon or evening. Our changed living conditions should make us think and raise our curiosity at the same time. It is important to ask the question of how dangerous our sun might really be. Would it not then be advisable for us to check on the reverse scenario? Are there perhaps risks involved in using all those highly marketed kinds of sun protection? How much money does the pharmaceutical industry make on us? Finally, is the sun not our enemy at all and the ozone hole not as dangerous as we think? Perhaps we all need a lot more of the precious warming good!

The fact is, sun protection products come with an enormous profit potential. The turnover for sun cosmetic care products in Germany alone rose to an annual volume of 129.8 million Euros until March 2010 due to research released by the Nielsen Market Research Company. The turnover in the United States of America regarding sun protection products had already reached over 300 million Dollars in the year 2005, whilst it remained relatively unknown in the 60s. The business with the sun grows just as rapidly as the skin cancer cases. For the coming years, the industry predicts an enormous growth potential in countries like India because of the fast-paced population growth. Whoever has just the slightest inkling of economic mechanisms will know that needs have to be created in order to increase consumer demand and, therefore, the turnover, as well as, the profit margins. Is it possible the sun is labeled as a scapegoat to increase the demands for sun screening products?

An important fact regarding the strength of the sun for a healthy life is very often overlooked. It concerns the production of vitamin D. Our body certainly needs the sun in order to produce sufficient vitamin D. It is desperately needed for the strengthening of our immune system and for the prohibition of carcinogenesis, influenza and infection. It assists in the prevention of developing depression, osteoporosis and it balances our hormones and many others. Meanwhile, research shows many people in industrialized nations suffer from a sun vitamin deficiency. For example, about 70 percent of the white population and 97 percent of the black population in the USA suffer from vitamin D deficiency.

The reason for this deficiency is not just due to people not spending enough time in the sun but also to insufficient nutrition. Unfortunately, during the past decades fast food chains have been on the steady rise. Our eating habits have changed for the worse, just like the quality of our food products. Our bodies do not get the substances needed any longer. For example, we should have a natural power of resistance against sunburn.

It is well known that sun protection from within affects us in the most natural manner. Therefore, we should consume antioxidant foods as much as possible. The so-called super foods are excellent providers of these. One supplementary substance is astaxanthin, which transports its lipophilic carothinoides into the skin cells. That way it protects the skin from UV-radiation. Therefore, it is possible for all of us to protect ourselves from sunburn, providing we consume a balanced diet and we take responsibility for the sensible exposure to our sun. To put it simply, a few cups of green tea for breakfast, some blueberries, salmon for lunch and a portion of carotene can be very useful. The truth is that UV-radiation can only cause skin cancer, if the UV-radiation works in conjunction with a chronic lack of a balanced nutrition. However, this is not widely communicated in the media, or by dermatologists and medical specialists, cancer research institutions, our health and safety departments or sunscreen producers. All we get to hear time and again is the importance of sunscreen products, protective clothes and sunglasses.

Dr. Alexander Wunsch, a German medical doctor and scientist specializing in the biology of light, points out the self-protection mechanisms within everybody. Our skin adapts naturally very well to the light exposure of our seasons. This, however, is a mechanism, which develops slowly over time following our biological clock. This natural process may lead to a sun protection factor of "50"within our skin. Yet, what happens in reality? People travel from one country to another in a matter of hours, very often to escape the winter months, and are surprised if they immediately catch sunburn. If handled in this way, our body does not have sufficient time to adapt to the radical change of sun exposure. The natural process, which is the best sun protection available, requires about 28 days to adapt.

The powers that deprive us of the fact that we carry the answer of sun protection within ourselves. Moreover, we are also being deprived of the fact that nearly all conventional sunscreen products contain chemicals that might lead to cancer. These are toxic chemical solvents containing oils decomposed from crude oil as well as artificial fragrances and strong alcohols. We should carefully consider the information and directions for use regarding the contents of toxic chemicals at all times. The list is long; such substances might be among others:

octyl salicylate, avobenzone, para aminobenzoic acid, oxybenzone, cinoxate, padimate o, dioxybenzone, phenylbenzimidazole, homosalate, sulisobenzone, methyl, anthranilate, trolamine salicylate, octocrylene.

Well that sounds like in a chemistry laboratory, perhaps you might find it easier to check for the following syllabics: ethyl…, butyl…, propyl…, methyl…, trieth… and dieth…, to name just a few.

When shopping for sun screen products it is always important to choose from the most natural products available and to make sure they contain no synthetic fragrances.

Ordinary sunscreen products often contain more than a dozen cancers causing chemical fragrances. By applying sunscreen, we rub the toxins into our skin. That way we strain our liver and the chances of developing cancer increases. Unfortunately, there are no warnings concerning possible health risks on the tubes, packages and tubs.

Australia even labels all alcoholic drinks with warning signs and it is one of the first countries to have banned advertising on cigarette packaging, but there are not yet any warnings on conventional sunscreens. Please avoid conventional synthetic sunscreens and preferably switch to the mineral-based ones. Please keep in mind synthetic sunscreens penetrate the skin, but they will not be completely absorbed by our body and will therefore linger in our organs.

A case study undertaken by the University of California could prove sun cream can damage the skin under certain circumstances. The UV-filters - octyl methoxycinnamate, benzophenone-3 and octocrylene, licensed in Germany quickly penetrate into the deep dermal layer. In next to no time all the protection for the upper layers is gone. Then the UV-filter substances quickly change to highly reactive oxygen compounds in the deeper tissue, which result in additional oxidative stress. That is exactly what we are trying to protect ourselves from. [11]

Other research points out that we should be cautious when handling sunscreens. On the one hand, they mislead us into thinking it is OK to stay in the sun for longer than is advisable because we think we are sufficiently protected by the sun cream, on the other hand, we seem to forget they do not protect us from skin cancer. The longer we expose ourselves to the sun the higher the doses of the UV-radiation and therefore the risk to develop melanomas. The opinion of newly released research states we should not expose ourselves to sun for any longer than we would without sunscreens. More detailed information can be found in the Journal of Clinical Oncology, Vol. 29, No 18 (June 20), 2011: pp e557-e558 and on the

internet pages:
http://www.destinationsante.com/Sun-cream-doesn-t-stop-cancer.html

Oliver Gillie, an experienced publisher of medical literature, accurately summarizes the facts on an example of Great Britain in one of the most extensive researches "Sunlight Robbery – Health benefits of sunlight are denied by current public health policy in the UK": "Active exposure of the skin to the sun by removing clothes and sunbathing is necessary to provide healthy levels of vitamin D… Vitamin D from nutrition provides only for 10 percent of our demand."*[12]*

He is trying to show us with his research how important it is for our health to expose ourselves to the sun on a regular basis. We need the sun to lead a healthy life. If we want to prevent cancer, it is essential to spend enough time in sunlight. The vitamin D obtained through nutrition is not sufficient for our body's demand, we need the additional strength of our sun. Even our nutrition does not have the required quality to provide for at least a minimum of our demand.

What really makes us sick are our modern and unrelated ways of living. It is fashionable to return from holidays deeply tanned; it cannot be brown enough, for our return from our well-earned break into our poor artificial environment. The sunbeds in our cities are used as substitutes - sunbeds without comprehensive user guidance and warnings. Over-tanned people sold to us as idols slime down at us in widespread advertisements. These idols usually use super creams. Consumer patterns concerning our sun for commercial purposes are created in this way.

Some of us think it is very cool to wear fashionable sunglasses. Yet, people have forgotten that sunglasses only turned fashionable in the thirties. Air force pilots wore them in various Hollywood movies. These movies became very popular and with them the sunglasses. Initially, special glasses were only known to people who displayed very sensitive reactions to sunlight. The birth of sunglasses actually dates back to the 7th century in China. Back then, quartz crystals were tinted. However, that was not done for the purposes of protection from the sun, but rather to conceal the eyes. These glasses were particularly famous with judges trying to hide their facial expressions.

So, why are we wearing sunglasses today? Most of think we have to wear them for UV-protection. For others, it is just a matter of style! Yet, nobody questions the side effects. Wearing glasses regularly has a significant impact on our natural rhythm. It is very important for our eyes to experience sunrises and sunsets in their natural light and appearance. It is important to be in balance with the rhythms of nature. By wearing darkened glasses, our natural synchronization fades very quickly and therefore our natural alignment between light and dark, i.e. day and night. Our eyes adapt to the light of the sun just as our skin does.

Allow your eyes to sunbathe regularly, meaning, with closed eyelids. This way your eyes will soon adapt to more intense light and any sensitivity to the light will be reduced. Dr. Jacob Liberman managed to prove that the regular use of sunglasses had a desensitizing effect on the photoreceptors in the eye, which led to an artificial intolerance of sunlight. He warns, in addition, sunglasses suppress important signals which alert us to exceptional brightness (For example, during a summer's day on the beach or during a sunny day in a skiing resort). Our eyes are very sensitive, and are able to distinguish between and adapt to light fluctuations. However, the regular use of sunglasses minimizes that natural alignment. Liberman says: "Should you have to wear sunglasses, change to a neutral grey coloration. Trend colors like yellow, pink, blue or red have extreme negative impacts on our eyes and might affect your health in another negative way." He is particularly concerned about children and babies wearing sunglasses. He urges not to use sunglasses on children, only in exceptional cases. "Today, we cannot foresee long term impacts of sunglasses on the development of a child. Tests showed it is important for eyes to visualize the entire spectrum of natural light (also UV-light), in order to promote an optimal development of the body."[13]

Isn´t it mainly our attitude, which makes us so vulnerable to eye diseases and skin cancer! It is the illusion of a quick, brown tan. Why is it not possible for us to simply interact with the sun in a manner that is in line with our nature? Nature has always been able to adapt to the sun. In hot countries like Spain, people have developed a long lunch break called a "Siesta". People work in the morning hours and again from the late afternoon onwards. People have always adapted and so have our animals. During the extreme midday heat in the savannas and steppes, animals search for shelter or dig themselves into the sand. The same accounts for us as well. The most affordable and ideal sun protection is shade. Just stay there during times of high sun-radiation. We can all sense when it is enough for our skin and eyes, so please simply move into a shady spot. Instead of blaming ozone holes and an omnipresent change in climate for our medical conditions, we should look to our own responsibility and nourish us with the precious attributes of our sun. We need the sun to stay healthy and our health should be our most valuable good.

4. The Healing Power of the Sun

A) Vitamin D, Life-Elixir

We have already learned something about vitamin D and we should take a closer look at its intensive protective mechanisms.

I would like to start with the definition of the term vitamin D, which is widely used in our colloquial language. This term is not entirely correct because vitamins are vital nutrients, which stem from substances outside our bodies. From the previous chapter we know however, we produce vitamin D with the assistance of our sun in our skin. Additionally, it is possible to gain vitamin D from our nutrition or through medication, but that cannot be equated with the sun. The vitamin D, which is generated from the sun in our skin as well the vitamin D intake via our nutrition, is called vitamin D3. Vitamin D3 is metabolized in the liver and from there, it supplies our body, something we will be able to observe on the consequential examples. Looking at the concept of vitamin D and its structures it becomes obvious it is more like a hormone, and in particular one of the steroid hormones. Part of that hormone group is cortisone and the sexual hormones. Therefore, it is better to use the term sun hormone from here on, instead of vitamin D.

In the past, the sun hormone was well known for its positive effect in relation to healthy teeth and strong bones. Today, we are aware of this being only the tip of the iceberg, as the sun hormone has a significant effect on our entire health. It is more significant than protecting our children from rickets and our elderly from osteoporosis. Many of our chronic diseases could be avoided by a sufficient intake of the sun hormone. It also strengthens our entire health and the whole of our immune system.

In that context, statistics concerning the deficiency of sun hormones in humankind are shocking. Research published in the European Journal of Clinical Nutrition in 2008 reports about a test conducted in 1998 on the German population namely, 1763 men and 2267 women aged between 18 and 79. On average, 57 percent of the men and 58 percent of all women suffered from a Vitamin D rate that was too low. Mainly, elderly women aged between 65 and 79 were affected. Of that group, about 75 percent showed a deficiency in vitamin D. [14]

Not only German adults are affected by a deficiency of sun hormones, children are as well. More than 17.000 children have been tested and they too showed a very intense lack of vitamin D. The deficiency during the summer months lay at a little lower than 50 percent compared to the winter when it rose to 60 percent.[15]

During the summer months, children play in the sun more often than in winter. Figures regarding the elderly population raise concern. In modern society, the elderly rarely live at home any longer but in old-age homes. Research shows that it is particularly those residents from nursing homes, who suffer from a deficiency of the sun hormone. The sun hormone deficiency in rest homes should be above 90 percent. It is therefore a significant factor in cardio vascular diseases, diabetes, cancer, osteoporosis, depression, kidney disease, thyroid disease, coordination disorder etc.

Not only research done in Germany shows significant deficiencies of the sun hormone, but also research completed in much more sun intensive countries like India and Australia. To a certain extent, it is true the sun hormone deficiency is dependent on the latitude and the seasons. However, it is also true that the living conditions in industrialized countries have changed. In fact, it does not matter in such countries how much sun there is available because the changed conditions of modern society take over and dictate how much sun we get to see despite the positive surrounding environment. As a result, there will be a deficiency.

For example, many people suffer from skin cancer in Australia. Many parents take this fact very seriously and tend to overprotect their children, which in turn can result in an acute vitamin D deficiency. These adults only allow their children to play outside if they are smothered in sun cream and wear a hat. In 2011, Australia was one of the first countries to propose legislation for regions of the country with less sun, such as South Australia and Tasmania. The directive says schoolchildren should play in the sun bareheaded for intervals of at least two hours several times a week, particularly during the winter months. Australia realized the sun is not only a risk factor for developing skin cancer but too little sun endangers the health of the young generations.

Spain, another sunny country, published a research paper from the Research Group in Valencia on May 19, 2011 in the Science Daily stating vitamin D from sun exposure protects children from asthma. The research, which had been conducted on 45,000 children and teenagers from nine Spanish cities, could prove that children from cooler and wetter cities run a higher risk of developing asthma.[16]

Supplying our bodies with the very important sun hormone has an extremely positive effect on our immune system. It adopts regulatory functions. If the immune system is too weak, then it will be stimulated. If it has strong reactions, as for instance in cases of rheumatism or inflammatory gastric diseases, the sun hormone displays the characteristic to regulate the overreaction of the immune system. Antibiotics naturally produced in the body will be stimulated and already penetrated bacteria and viruses can be fought off.[17]

Furthermore, the sun hormone regulates the autoimmune process in Type I diabetes. In this disease, the immune defense destroys the insulin producing cells of the pancreas. Yet, the hormone also assists in cases of Type II diabetes, which reflect an insulin resistance. Research from the University of Melbourne, Australia has shown a significant lower risk to develop Type II diabetes in people with sufficient vitamin D levels. Over 5,000 people were tested over a period of five years. The tests indicate people with lower than average vitamin D levels run a 57 times higher risk of developing Type II diabetes. Prof. Peter Ebeling, employee of the Western Health Services, explained the research findings in a TV-interview with the Australian ABC in July 2011. He explained, as soon as the vitamin D level dropped in a patient, the risk of developing the disease increased. If we were to decrease the daily dose of vitamin D by 25 units, would it then be the case that the risk of Type II diabetes was to increase by 24 percent? In sunny regions of Australia 10 minutes of sun exposure in summer every day before 10 am and after 2pm and in winter for about 30 minutes respectively should be sufficient to satisfy our demand of vitamin D.[18] Yet about a third of the population in a sunny country like Australia suffers from vitamin D deficiency.

Furthermore, the sun hormone has an influence on our nervous system and controls the improvement of the teamwork between nerves and muscles. Our coordination improves and we fall less often. Sufficient sun exposure additionally increases bone density and therefore avoids osteoporosis and the risks involved in falling. With these arguments in mind, we should have the heart to spend some time in sunlight during the winter months and escape from the so often diagnosed winter depression in countries like Germany. The German Weather Bureau (Deutscher Wetterdienst) announced on the February 27, 2013 that Germany had a total of 96 hours of sunshine on average during the winter of 2012/13 as well as from the beginning of December 2012 until the end of February 2013 and therefore experienced the darkest winter since the beginnings of nationwide meteorological data recording in the year 1951. These findings can be stated based on the results of 2000 monitoring stations. An average German winter has about 154 sunny hours, which is still very little.

To sum up, it can be said that our general health will improve with the assistance of the sun hormone. In particular, people who cannot expose themselves to the sun for cultural reasons - like women wearing a veil and clothes concealing their whole body due to religion, - should take supplements. Furthermore, all shift workers and people in nursing homes should have their sun hormone levels checked. Professor Peter Ebeling advises the additional intake of supplements for these population groups.

It would however be sensible to restore your need for vitamin D from nature directly. The business regarding vitamin D supplements has grown to a million dollar business. The German magazine "Das Ärzteblatt" published in January 2014 stated that the turnover in the USA concerning vitamin D supplements has risen from 42 million US-Dollars in 2002 to 605 million US-Dollars in 2011, which constitutes a tenfold increase.

We should ask the question - how much vitamin D is necessary?

My research resulted in unbelievably large tolerances within globally published statistics. One explanation is the sun hormone has not been very popular until a short time ago and scientists assumed much lower minimum levels. However, recently released research shows contrasting results with much higher units. The aforementioned Australian research recommends a daily minimum unit of 600 IU. A doctor from the University of Miami, Silvana Lewis recommends 1,000 to 2,000 units, 800 units should be sufficient but if a patient suffers from a chronic illness, more is advisable. Dieter Felsenberg, an expert on muscle and bone disorders at the Charité in

Berlin supports this opinion. Other sources refer to 4,000 IU per day in order to ensure sufficient care for the body cells. In particular, pregnant women need higher levels of the sun hormone, in order to care for their babies.

Furthermore, the terms I.E., IU and µg are very confusing. The conversion factor between units reads as follows:

1µg (microgram) = 40 I.U. (International Units). The abbreviation for I.E. is the German version (Internationale Einheiten) and stands for I.U. 1 µg leads to an increase in the blood of 1nmol/l.

Well, if our demand for sun hormones is enormously high, the next question of how can we cater for such a demand must inevitably follow.

- Spending a modest and regular time in the sun
- Via our nutrition (see chart)
- The additional intake of supplements (this should be done in consultation with a doctor)

In as far as nutrition goes, we can easily rely on fish, as it contains the highest percentage of vitamin D:

Recommended fish types and other foods are:

Foods	concentration per 100 g in µg
Herring	31
Salmon	16.3
Eel	13
Tuna	5.4
Halibut	5
Button mushroom	1.9
Ox liver	1.7

This statistic is only a selection of vitamin D rich foods. Of course, other foods like butter, eggs, avocados and cows' milk contain the sun hormone as well.

At this point we need to ask ourselves another question – Is it possible to overdose on the sun hormone?

In standard practice, the answer is yes however, it is highly unlikely to overdose because the intake through foods makes up only about 10 percent of our demand of the sun hormone. Only the consumption of too much cod liver oil could lead to an overreaction but I think the bad taste will do the trick in protecting us from an overdose. When it comes to supplements, it is always wise to consult a doctor because, as mentioned before, a therapeutic effect might only result from a very high dose and should be monitored professionally. It is important to have the relevant blood tests done.

In general, there are no known side effects from a too high dose. However, should symptoms like tiredness thirst, nausea, feeling faint and headaches persist, it is advisable to consult a doctor of your trust in any case.

B) Sun against Cancer

Several current studies show a correlation between the sun hormone and a variety of cancers like bowel cancer, breast cancer, prostate cancer, skin cancer, lung cancer and other cancerous tumors.

Evidently, significant research shows in most cases the chance of developing cancer could be reduced with raised vitamin D levels in the blood or that men and women with higher sun hormone levels are at a lower risk of developing cancerous diseases.

Bowel Cancer:

Annually about 70,000 people fall ill due to bowel cancer and about 30,000 people die from it every year.[19] Hence, Germany ranks number one in the global comparison.[20]

The risk of developing bowel cancer rises steadily from the age of fifty onwards. According to information of the Robert-Koch-Institute in Berlin, the average age in men to develop bowel cancer is about 69 years and in women about 75 years. To minimize countries at risk, like Germany and Australia, bowel (blood) tests from the age of 50 are now offered free of charge. Another preventative method is the colonoscopy also called prevention colonoscopy. Apart from nutritional habits and exercise, the most effective prevention is the sun hormone, which even today is only little communicated! This is despite the proof of many researches, which confirmed the important effects on our wellbeing concerning our bowel.

First, consolidated findings came from a geographical date concerning cancer. People living in sunnier latitudes are at a significantly lower risk at developing a disease like bowel cancer than people who experience less sun exposure.

The cancer atlas referring to the USA shows a significantly higher mortality rate from bowel cancer in the North West compared to the South East.[21] Scientists have discovered that the South East has more hours of sunshine and have combined the different data.

Another research resulted in similar findings. This time the research came from a European region and was undertaken by Professor Johan Moan and his team at the Institute for Cancer Research in Oslo, Norway. It states the chances for survival when diagnosed with bowel cancer are significantly higher, if diagnosed in summer or autumn in contrast to diagnoses in or straight after a "vitamin D-winter", when all the "stored" vitamin D-reserves are used or are highly minimized.[22]

Additionally, a different analysis is very interesting; about 85,000 men and 105,000 women on Hawaii and in California aged above 45 years replied to extensive questionnaires concerning their habits and nutrition between 1993 and 1996. Recently, scientists from the Universities of Honolulu and Southern-California have utilized data from this resource to find answers to the question about the importance of calcium and vitamin D regarding bowel cancer. The result confirmed the findings of many other studies from previous years: "Calcium and vitamin D, in particular, their typical interaction, has a significant influence on the risk to develop bowel cancer."[23]

To put all the studies and research briefly, it can be said that all of those findings point to one and the same result namely; sufficient vitamin D in our bodies reduces the risk of developing bowel cancer or respectively increases the chances of healing. What process is taking place in our body and can the sun hormone be useful as a method of therapy for bowel cancer?

A Spanish Research Team asked exactly that question and discovered a complex mutual reaction: "The active biologic form of vitamin D (1a, 25-dihydroxyvitamin D3) activates in turn a gen, which stimulates a protein by the name of Cystatin D. This protein suppressed at least during laboratory experiments the growth of colon cancer cells. The cancer cells divided less frequently, lost their flexibility and switched off genes which promoted the growth of cancer."[24]

It is not just in the context with bowel cancer that the sun hormone has a very positive effect on our health. It also shows correlations in many other types of cancerous diseases.

Breast Cancer:

Most incidences of cancer are reported in regards to women in Germany as well as in Europe. During the year 2008, a total of 27.8 percent of all cancerous diseases in women in Germany related to breast cancer. Annually, about 17,500 women will die from this illness. The average age to develop the disease stands at 63.[25] Mainly women aged between fifty-five and seventy are diagnosed with breast cancer.

In Europe the incidences are estimated at 350,000 whilst 130,000 will die as a result. Therefore, breast cancer is accountable for 26. 5 percent of all cancerous diseases and for 17.5 percent of all causes of death relating to cancer in Europe's adult female population.[26]

According to information from the American Cancer Society, the estimated figure referring to incidences related to breast cancer is at 178,480 for the year 2007. The WHO sadly expects globally more than half a million women will die as a result of breast cancer every year.[27]

The report on mamma-carcinoma-risk factors also named MARIE published in 2009 – study, shows a significant correlation between vitamin D and breast cancer. This case study on the causes of breast cancer after the menopause was conducted on 11,054 women, 3,813 of whom were diagnosed with breast cancer between 2002 and 2005. The women were questioned in regards to hormone therapies, lifestyle and environmental factors. In addition to the questionnaires on nutrition, blood samples were collected and examined. In order to analyze the correlation between vitamin D and breast cancer, the vitamin D drawn from nutrition or the total vitamin D level including the internal syntheses, measured in the blood has to be taken into account. Since the research already detected a correlation between vitamin D from nutrition and the risk to develop breast cancer, it was decided to take an additional approach regarding all women's vitamin D status (25-hydroxy-vitamin-D-level in blood). About half of all research participants had a vitamin D level below 50nmol/l, which is seen as a minimal Vitamin D deficiency in the long run. The patients had a substantial lower vitamin D level compared to the healthy women. A decrease in the risk of breast cancer could be noted when the vitamin D levels increased.[28]

Therefore, vitamin D is not only important in conjunction with the calcium balance and the bone structures but also in regards to its cancer restraining characteristics as shown by the regulation of cell growth and cell division.

Further research on the prevention of breast cancer was published in the magazine "The Journal of Steroid Biochemistry and Molecular Biology; 103(3-5):708-1 in March 2007. Reports on the internet state research findings regarding women being less at risk of developing breast cancer if they have the highest serum levels of vitamin D (25-hydroxyvitamin D) in their blood. Furthermore, it is said that a daily intake of 2,000 I.U. (International Units) of vitamin D3 and about 12 minutes of sun exposure (during midday, without sun protection/depending on season and location) daily will take the vitamin D level to a high of (serum 25(OH)D), which is the value at which breast cancer cases are reduced to about 50 percent.[29]

Similarly fascinating results were published in The American Journal of Clinical Nutrition on 14th of April 2010. Reuter's states, with reference to this scientific report, the risk of developing breast cancer in women can be reduced by 24 percent with a dose of at least 400 I.U. (International Units) of vitamin D.[30]

Further reports on that topic come from Mr. Slevin in Australia, who is co-author of a report in The Medical Journal of Australia and speaker of The Cancer Counsel in Australia. The report says two to six minutes of sun exposure during the lunch break in spring and summer about three to four times a week will suffice for absorbing the recommended vitamin D level in our body.[31]

It can be concluded, the higher the vitamin D level the lower the risk to develop breast cancer.

Prostate Cancer:

The most frequently diagnosed type of cancer in men is prostate cancer. In second and third place are bowel and lung cancer. The high frequency particular in industrial nations is noticeable. It mostly affects men at over 65 years of age. The estimated global cases in men diagnosed with prostate cancer stand at 678,000.[32] According to estimates, one in five men will develop this disease during his life span.[33]

Due to statistics on early diagnoses of prostate cancer, it became interestingly obvious that men from North America developed just as often prostate cancer as men from Europe, but the progression of the disease was less likely to occur. Therefore, a correlation between it and nutrition is assumed. Further findings might show that prostate cancer was more often diagnosed in regions with less sunshine. We already know from the chapters on other cancerous diseases, vitamin D is activated by sunlight in our skin and is therefore important for cell differentiation. The absorption of vitamin D could have a certain protective effect.[34]

When positively diagnosed with the disease, the immediate therapy is usually concentrated on observation, an operation, radiation-, or hormone therapy. To date, vitamin D does not have a significant component of any form of therapy. So far, health professionals have very opposing opinions concerning the treatment of prostate cancer. Some simply prefer to do nothing, others want to observe, whilst others take the stand it is best to remove the cancer as soon as possible in an early stage.

However, it is certain that the figure regarding annually positively diagnosed cases increases steadily. There are several explanations for this. One might be the ever-improving cancer screening and early diagnoses, the other might sadly be the changed living habits of modern society in industrialized communities. According to statistics from the Robert Koch Institute, incidences in Germany have doubled between the years of 1980 and 2006. The German Cancer Research Institute published diverse results from a Meta-Analysis on the topic of vitamin D and prostate cancer. The results could not show a significant correlation. However, a scientific research team from the USA at the Midwestern Regional Medical Center, Zion, II (Cancer Treatment Center of America) took the trouble to abstract all-important research results on the topic of vitamin D and the risk of developing prostate cancer because it was suspected there might be a correlation between prostate cancer and vitamin D.

April 7, 2009 saw the release of an online report stating that seven studies showed little or no correlation between the disease and the sun hormone. However, ten research studies published between the years of 1992 and 2008 showed the significant effect the sun hormone has on the illness. It became very obvious a lot of research still has to be done in this respect.

In the year 2006, the European Journal of Cancer published an article from the Netherlands with the title: "Does Sunlight prevent cancer? A systematic Review"[35] It is stated that all eight related research studies showed the existence of a proportional correlation between the chances of falling ill with prostate cancer or even dying from it and sunlight. A quantitative correlation between sunlight and the mortality rate of prostate cancer obviously follows a dose-effect-graph: "the prevention becomes more effective when more sunlight is absorbed."[36] [37]

More recent research published in 2010 coming from the United States, conducted by the scientists Omar Flores and Kerry L. Burnstein from the Department of Molecular and Cellular Pharmacology, University of Miami Miller School of Medicine, 1600 NW 10th Avenue, Miami, Florida 33136, engages in the correlation between genes and the sun hormone.

The subject of the sun and prostate cancer becomes increasingly interesting and further research results can be expected in the near future.

The correlation between the sun hormone and prostate cancer can no longer be questioned. Ongoing research promises exciting results.

C) The Sun during Pregnancy

The count of the world's population at present stands at 7,128,178,612 people living on our planet Earth. Annually, the world's population grows by about 82,947,000 people, with 227,252 per day, 158 per minute and 2.6 humans per second.[38]

Germany is amongst the countries with the lowest population growth. Due to statistics published by the Federal Office for Statistics of the Federal Republic of Germany, 677,947 babies were born alive in Germany in the year 2010. Stillbirths came to 2,466 and 2,322 children had died during their first year of life.[39]

We should be very aware of such figures because the health of our mothers and children is at stake. Again, it becomes apparent; vitamin D is an important role player in this context.

During pregnancy, a mother-to-be does not only carry the responsibility for herself but also for the growing baby. The effect of vitamin D on bone structure and teeth (adamantine) during pregnancy regarding the unborn child is common knowledge. In order to protect the healthy development of the baby's teeth every gynecologist will question moms-to-be about a sufficiently milk product rich diet. However, the role vitamin D plays in this is only very rarely explained. A vitamin D deficiency can lead to early miscarriages and other disorders.

It is furthermore known, people whose mothers had sufficient vitamin D in their blood during their own childhood or during pregnancy, face a lower risk of developing multiple scleroses. An article called "Vitamin D – the gate to heaven" (article 394 dd. 04.01.2010) reports about Prof. B. Tayler (Hobart) research on 145 multiple scleroses patients. He states, "… increasing vitamin D levels in the blood arrange for less relapses. More accurately: for every increase of 10nmol of vitamin D, the risk to suffer from a new relapse decreased by 10 percent. Was the vitamin D level in the blood doubled, the risk to experience another relapse halved."[40]

Similar results can be read about in regards to osteoporosis. A survey conducted by the British Medical Research Council shows that children whose mothers took vitamin D supplements during pregnancy had a higher bone density at the age of nine compared to other children. The results as published in the Lancet (2006; 367:36-43) raise the question about an increase in vitamin D supplements during pregnancy.

Further correlations between pregnancy and vitamin D were looked into. A research article with the title "Correlation between vitamin D3 deficiency and insulin resistance in pregnancy" reports on 741 pregnant women, 70.6 percent of who suffered from vitamin D deficiency. The results showed an obvious correlation between the vitamin D levels and insulin resistance in pregnancy. Other studies assume another correlation between vitamin D and type II diabetes.[41]

Respiratory infections in newborns as well are linked to vitamin D levels in mothers and babies. For that reason, newborn babies in Turkey have received 400I.U. of vitamin D supplements from the Health Ministry since 2005 per day during the first year of living. Long ago, Turkey discovered the correlation between the health of newborns and vitamin D. Additionally, Turkey conducts research on infections of the lower respiration tract. Sixteen boys and nine girls were monitored, as well as, a control group of six boys and nine girls. The babies were the same regarding birth weight, length, head size and age. All babies were breast-fed and no premature infants were amongst the group. The vitamin D levels of all mothers were listed and a significant correlation between the vitamin D level of the moms and their babies was detected. Was the vitamin D level found to be low in the mother, it was also low in the baby. Yet, the results showed another correlation as well. Babies with low vitamin D faced an increased risk of developing an infection of the lower respiration tract.[42]

I want to do without any further research on mothers and children in connection with the vitamin D at this point because I think the examples above made the importance of a sufficiently high vitamin D level during pregnancy very clear. The obvious answer here is the child will always be like its mother. If a healthy development for the child is to be achieved, it is important that the mother takes all precautions. Vitamin D is certainly not the only thing that has to be taken care of during pregnancy. Smoking and alcohol consumption have to be minimized or stopped, the folic acid has to be monitored just like the omega 3 fatty acid and many other issues have to be considered. Pregnant women should always consult a health professional. This chapter wants to show the importance of the mother's health and wellbeing during pregnancy has on the child's entire course of life.

If there is a deficiency of the fetus during pregnancy, the baby will be born with deficiencies, which might develop into diseases during the maturing person's entire course of life. Therefore, every woman should be very conscious during pregnancy and breast feeding concerning healthy nutrition.

If the mother's metabolism is not adequately supplied, it might affect the entire future of the child and that means not only deficiencies and disorders but also the functions of its genes. The nine months of pregnancy are thus extremely responsible for the newborn's entire course of life. If the mother is not adequately supplied with vitamin D during the pregnancy, it might quickly lead to diabetes, high blood pressure or even to premature birth. Premature birth may lead to other high risks, which might have an influence on the brain function of the child during its lifespan.

Furthermore, children whose mothers have had normal pregnancies, yet a depleted supply of vitamin D run a higher risk of developing diseases like diabetes or osteoporosis in their lifetime. Very often, the immune system will not be strong enough to protect them from infections or allergies and the genes, as well as, their receptors might be changed. The list is long and a lot of research is still required. Furthermore, there is a significant need for more education regarding pregnancies in order to assure a continued healthy human race. Vitamin D and our sun are major stakeholders in regards to our health.

Please note: If a pregnant woman is adequately supplied with vitamin D, the baby will be as well and that has a positive effect on the course of the pregnancy, the newborn as well as the further lifespan of the child.

D) Cardiovascular Disease

Due to reports published by the Federal Office for Statistics in Wiesbaden, Germany in December 2012 - cardiovascular diseases are the most likely cause of death. More than 40 percent of all deaths during 2011 were due to a cardiovascular disease. About 92 percent of all people concerned were 65 years of age or older. A total of 145,500 men and 196,600 women died from cardiovascular disease in Germany during 2011. Global statistics show a significantly higher percentage of people succumbing to cardiovascular disease in western industrialized nations. The global figure of people suffering from cardiovascular problems is estimated at 22 million. The most likely cardiovascular diseases are coronary heart diseases, stroke and heart attack. Heart attack on its own with over 60,000 fatalities annually in Germany is the second most common cause for death. Widely spread risk factors for developing a cardiovascular disease are high blood pressure, stress, being overweight, alcohol, smoking and lack of exercise.

In that respect, we should look at some interesting research concerning vitamin D as we have done in the previous chapters.

According to current studies, vitamin D deficiency is linked to an increased risk of developing a stroke, heart attack, arterial occlusion and the heart's pumping action possibly being too weak.

Prof. Dr. Armin Zittermann abstracts in his article "Vitamin D and its importance in preventive medicine" numerous interesting aspects. "Large scale prospective and not randomized studies like the LURIC study in Germany and the Hoorn study in the Netherlands could conclude a deficient vitamin D supply is in general and in particular an independent risk factor in cardiovascular mortality and in deadly strokes, unexpected heart death and death caused by heart insufficiency ... A Meta analyses of randomized, prospective studies showed during a follow up period of 5.7 years the total mortality in persons middle-aged and old-aged could be reduced by 7 percent by a low dose of supplementation of vitamin D (10 to 20 μg daily)." He reports furthermore, "The Framingham-Offspring-Study could show people with 25-hydroxyvitamin D levels lower than 37.5 nmol/l run a 4.4 times higher risk of developing a cardiovascular event within the next 5 years compared to people with better vitamin D levels. Vitamin D has positive effects on important cardiovascular risk factors. Available Meta analyses show vitamin D deficiency correlates with an increased risk of diabetes mellitus and that additional vitamin D supplementation can significantly lower the blood pressure."[43]

The German Center for Diabetes in Düsseldorf reports that the risk to develop a cardiovascular disease in diabetics with vitamin D deficiency is double that in healthy people. Carlos Bernal-Mizrachi and colleague staff members of the Washington University School of Medicine, St. Louis reported in an article published in the "Circulation" Magazine about the mechanisms in cardiovascular diseases regarding diabetes patients and vitamin D deficiency. In this context, the cholesterol in particular was checked because it was found that diabetics with vitamin D deficiency could not process the cholesterol correctly. Bernal-Mizrachi comments: "In people with vitamin D deficiency the macrophages will eat more cholesterol, but can´t absorb it. The cholesterol oversaturated macrophages will agglutinate and develop into the so called "foam cells" which are a first sign of arteriosclerosis." [44]

In this way, the bad cholesterol settles in the arteries, which subsequently narrow and the risk for a stroke or heart attack increases. The interesting part of this research is vitamin D can potentially stop the formation of foam cells.

Vitamin D and cardiac insufficiency are also in correlation. During the cause of cardiac insufficiency, inflammation supporting substances will be excessively released due to the illness. Stefanie Schulze Schleithoff managed to prove in her doctorate that patients showed an increase in inflammation inhabiting substances in the blood that, in turn, will lead to the suppression of inflammation supporting substances when supplemented with vitamin D.

Luckily, many more studies could be listed. Yet, in a nutshell, vitamin D plays a very significant role in the matter of cardiovascular diseases. Enough vitamin D assists the immune system, helps to lower cholesterol, lowers the blood pressure and should be more frequently discussed between health professionals and their patients concerning prevention. In that respect, many other factors are important and recommended together with the intake of numerous vitamins, minerals, natural micronutrients and omega 3 acid. An Exercise Physiologist from Brisbane, Australia told me about the importance of exercises in regards to the prevention of diseases.[45] Therefore, a good piece of advice might be to plan a sunny walk during your lunch break to a fish restaurant. The power of our sun influences our well-being on large scale.

Despite earlier awarded Nobel Prizes in science regarding vitamin D in the years of 1903 and 1928 the question whether we still have an enormous need for clarification needs to be asked. During the past years, the health profession is more devoted toward that topic. A desirable outcome would be an extensive clarification directed at the people on the fact of vitamin D syntheses in our bodies. Our generation has sadly been engaged with a conception that describes our sun as an enemy. This is a huge mistake with fatal consequences.

Please note: Vitamin D has positive effects concerning cardiovascular risk factors. It is important for prevention and the healing process.

5. Alternative Healing Methods of our Sun

A) The Sun's Healing Power as a part of Nature

Jacob Lorber (born July 22, 1800 in Kanischa, at the time Herzogtum Steiermark, died August 24, 1864 in Graz) coined the expression 'sun remedy' (German, Sonnenheilmittel). Jacob Lorber called himself http://www.hongkiat.com/blog/futuristic-home-furnitures/a "writing servant of God" because of his many intuitions, which he brought to paper. The violinist and author had many mystical experiences during his lifetime. Besides other very interesting themes, he was always dedicated to the research into sun remedies. Some of those are sunlight enriched natural products and heliopathy. He published a book with the title "The healing power of sunlight" as early as 1851 describing how sun energy could be locked onto agents like minerals, plants and animal based substances. He was absolutely convinced of the idea that the soul and therefore our body are benefiting from the sunlight agents during the healing process.

To date, many companies still produce sun remedies based on Jacob Lorber's traditional recipes. In order to explore how these sun remedies are made and what we should ask for, I visited some naturopathic practices. The remedies are available as cosmetics (to apply the skin or to rub in) or as dietary supplements. The sun globules seem to lead the way because they are supposed to carry the whole of the light spectrum in equal parts. The storage containers for the globules are very important. Thousands of years ago, people already discovered that it was best to store ointments and oils, etc. in violet colored containers. Even today, mainly violet colored jars are used to store sun remedies. The jars protect from diverse exposure to light and that way they will extend the shelf life. The globules are said to have a positive impact on moods. Another typical sun remedy is poppy flower oil. To produce this oil a mixture of poppy flower petals and olive oil is exposed to the sun for several weeks. The result is an ointment, which offers relieve from joint – and muscle pain.

Arnica lotion is a recommended remedy for skin irritation,

eczemas, lichen and atopic dermatitis. The remedy is made out of some arnica petals mixed with alcohol, which are then exposed to the sun for several weeks.

Juniper berries are used to detoxify, as an antiseptic and to assist with the release of water. They are recommended by naturopathies to combat contagious diseases. The collected wild berries are spread onto a linen sheet and exposed to the sun to obtain best results.

Other interesting sun remedies are chestnut powder, which is said to improve the blood values, camphor milk powder that is supposed to have a positive effective on the respiratory system, rhubarb power that strengthens the nerves and the bowel, sea salt, which is used in connection with a healthy bone structure, and many more ranging from hair growth oils to cures for tooth problems.

Should you have an interest in such substances I would recommend you visit a naturopath in your area or read more about sun remedies "Sonnenheilmittel" on the internet?

Despite the knowledge of observational research into sun remedies, they have been widely ignored by science and remain largely unexplored.

B) Heliotherapy

Heliotherapy is understood as a therapeutic method for humans harnessing the assistance of light rays and is known as light therapy.

This context brings us back to the work of Jacob Lorber. Yet, even long before his studies, mankind knew about the healing powers of light. It was practiced in ancient Greece and during the Egyptian time.

In the year 1903 the Danish Prof. Dr. Niels Rynberg Finsen received a Nobel Prize for his scientific studies concerning the use of light therapy. During the past 25 years light therapy has finally developed into a source of interest in Germany.

We learned in the previous chapter it is possible to absorb sunlight via cosmetics and food, which have been exposed to and therefore enriched with all the frequencies and light quanta of the sunlight. During the process of light therapy, full spectrum light is used with intense luminosity. This process involves filtering out UV- and infrared particles. This way the body can also be exposed to sufficient light during the European autumn – and winter months, which would be mostly impossible via the use of natural sunlight during those months.

Usually, patients will sit every day for about one to two weeks for a set amount of time in front of a light apparatus. It is, of course, easier, if sufficient sunlight is present in your region because this will ensure everybody will be able to enjoy the warmth of the sun directly on the whole body. However, please keep in mind such a highly effective balmy sunbaths should be used by keeping a sensible dosage in mind, so please do not get sun burned.

Sunbathing was mainly used to cure tuberculosis until the discovery of antibiotics. Today, mood swings as well as the winter depression are being healed with the assistance of our sun. In addition, skin diseases like psoriasis and eczemas form part of the therapy program.

Light transfers its positive powers onto our body, soul and spirit and therefore our whole wellbeing.

C) Chronobiology

What is chronobiology and what does it have to do with our sun?

Let us get started with the definition taken from the naturopathy lexicon, where chronobiology is defined as follows: "the doctrine of the rhythm in the organism. Our daily rhythm consists of sleep and hours of being awake. These are accompanied by other rhythms, which release for examples hormones adjusted to the daytime. The chronobiology has an important role to play during flights (Jetlag – tiredness after long distance flights due to changes in the rhythm) and in the astronautics."[46]

However, not only the daily rhythm between sunrise and sunset and vice versa but also the seasons and the phase of the moon need to be investigated in this context.

Chronobiology is a wide term and we could also understand it in the sense of studying our entire biorhythm.

Spring fever and winter depression, as well as, medication, which take better effect if taken at particular times of the day, are part of those studies.

And once again, the sun comes into play. The rhythm of light and dark is one of the important engines running in the background of human existence. However, this natural rhythm is progressively disrupted by our modern ways of life. For example, technical progress expects increased working patterns involving shift work. The destructive power of man's greed and globalization as well as the anxiety over losing one's job increases the extra hours at the work place rapidly. The jobs are often in office blocks or production halls with bad lighting and poor quality of light. Managers are jetting across several time zones around the globe against their inner clock. Races like this will have severe impacts. It will result in chronic diseases. These illnesses will burden the budget of our medical systems and therefore us taxpayers. And that is where the circle closes because we have arrived back at the light, which regulates our rhythms.

People in the modern society spend a lot of time in rooms with comparatively poor light quality. The average lighting inside is about 50 to 500 lux. Outside, it would be between 8.000 and 100.000 lux. You can see the enormous difference. Light is the most important factor in our time management but we barely pay any attention to it. Our body reacts only from 1.000 lux and above by being activated by the light as a rhythm engine. This engine is the power that lies behind our driving force and endurance. Just imagine the consequences for the masses of people, who spend almost their whole life below the 1.000 lux. Sleeping disorder, loss of energy, mood swings and depression are the fatal results.

Please read more about our light in the chapter about sunlight and artificial lighting.

Our body not only stores information about the daily routine but also about the seasons. Our new lifestyles sensitively disrupt this natural cycle. You should therefore not be surprised about your spring fever or winter depression; these are very natural processes.

Chronobiology is very well aware by now that every person has an individual set up in regards to their personal inner clock.

Early birds and night owls are regulated by hormones. If the inner clock works against the work shift, working hours, and the University - or school visit physical symptoms might easily occur just like a lack in concentration. It might therefore be a positive thing for late risers to get started a little later with their daily routine whilst early birds might find it difficult to be active and concentrate in the late evening hours.

It is hoped the research into chronobiology in all of those events and will gain more significance in the near future. The times of the day and rhythms are currently not really used in the diagnostics of disease patterns.

It is even worse for elderly people because the rhythm fades with increasing age. However, in fact people are getting older than ever in our societies and should therefore have the right to spend enough time in adequate light in order to stay healthy. Statistics are available concerning our aging population but there are no statistics available about sufficient lighting quality or sunshine for the elderly.

I picture an old age home facility in the municipality of Miesbach, Bavaria in Germany. That region is very close to the Alps and therefore has only a limited amount of sunshine hours and very long lasting, grey and dark winters.

The new facility was built directly adjacent to the main street in 2008, without a park, or walkways and without sun decks. This home for the elderly is only one of so many examples of concrete bunkers that keep the older generation hidden away behind walls. There is a very different approach in Australia or even South Africa. The so-called retirement villages are beautiful small villages where elderly people, who are in need of assistance, or company, or do not manage to maintain their larger estates any longer, are able to relax. These senior villages are located in sunny areas where every house has its own small garden and the walkways and parking lots are spacious. Retirees having problems walking are very often seen in small electric cars. These villages are close to medical facilities, meals can be provided for and usually, the shopping facilities are within reach. Furthermore, these houses are reasonably priced and they offer enough space and comfort for visitors as well. The elderly with an average and low income can only dream about such facilities in Germany. Investors who tried to introduce these ideas practiced in South Africa to Germany have previously been instantly scared away by the responsible authorities like municipalities and by politics.

Another certain way to disrupt our bio-rhythm dramatically is the idea of summer, – and winter time the so called day light savings.

In Germany, the clock is switched once during October and again in March. Besides all the little technical hiccups, our body is instantly thrown out of its natural rhythm. A Swedish research team conducted a study and found the time switch into summer time has massive consequences for humans.

It is alleged the risk of developing heart disease increases during that time due to lack of sleep. Not just humans are affected by the re-setting, animals as well. Local farmers report from Upper Bavaria their cows produce less milk in the immediate days after the change in time. The farmers say it takes several weeks before the cows adapt to the new time frames. This is different for farmers in Queensland, Australia because in that region, where farms are enormous measuring several hundreds of square kilometers, the population decided against day light savings.

It does not matter what efforts humans make to change our living conditions, it will be futile because nature cannot be dictated. Our metabolism, the kidney function, our concentration and our nervous system are linked to the rhythm of the day. It is the same for humans, animals and plants. I am thinking in particular about the day and night active animals as well as plants that coordinate their blossoms, fragrances and the nectar periodically during the day.

More detail on this topic is available in the chapters about photosynthesis and chlorophylls.

On October 24, 2007 an online report was published on Landlive.de with the title "Chronobiology: Every time switch tumbles our inner clock". The article reports about findings by Prof. Till Ronneberg at the Ludwig-Maximilians-University (LMU), Munich, who managed to show that switching the time has a more dramatic impact than previously suspected.

The inner clock dictates several behavior patterns in humans and many other processes in the body in predetermined cycles. This genetically provided mechanism synchronizes itself in this process with the environment – sunlight is the main "timer". Our inner clock adjusts with the assistance of daylight to a 24-hour-rhythm of the environment. Dawn is very important during this process, namely the change from night to day. Our sleep rhythm adapts to the time flow of the dawn from East to West within a time zone. The scientists utilized data from questionnaires in which they questioned about 55,000 people. The result stated, "The inner clock adapts to seasonal variations of the morning dawn", so Ronneberg. "During winter it is set on late and during summer on early. This minute adjustment is sensitively disturbed by daylight saving."[47]

Melatonin looms large in this context. Melatonin is a very important hormone, which regulates not only our day rhythm but also our daily routine and controls therefore our food intake and body temperature. The same accounts for fish, reptiles, amphibians and birds. Here, the melatonin production is regulated via the central nerve system, meaning within the visual scope. Our wristwatch cannot escape nature's time during the artificial introduction of summer - and winter times because there is no better synchronization impulse for our inner clock than sunlight.

About 20 percent of the light entering our eyes will be used for visualization. The remaining 80 percent regulate biological functions in our body. About 10 percent of the light impulses reach the pineal gland via the eye, optical nerve, and hypothalamus. Its most important function is the production of melatonin because with the assistance of day light it is possible to generate the very important serotonin from the amino acid tryptophan. As soon as the light impulses are gone, as e.g. during darkness, serotonin, also widely known as "happy hormone", changes into melatonin (sleep hormone).

This very sensitive process is highly dependent on natural light. If our body does not generate sufficient serotonin as e.g. in winter or due to bad artificial lighting or if we spend too little time outside, does this mean the melatonin will be affected? As mentioned before, melatonin on its behalf regulates our sleeping, waking, rhythm. Our melatonin levels are many times higher during nighttime than during the day and thus insure a healthy sleep.

Artificial light disrupts the production severely. Health professionals very often blame sleeping disorders on melatonin levels that are too low. A healthy sleep is important in order to maintain the necessary memory capacity in our day-to-day life. Melatonin is not only important in this context but also concerning the ductless glands and therefore our thyroids, pituitary glands, thymus, adrenal glands, gonadal and pancreas. It also plays an essential role for our growth, immune system, blood pressure, heartbeat, respiration, body temperature, digestion, osmoregulation etc.

Serotonin on the other hand is responsible for our mood. A low serotonin level can cause anxiety disorders, aggressions as well as, depressions. It has furthermore an impact on our cardiovascular system, our whole nerve system and the gastrointestinal tract.

Overweight people very often suffer from a serotonin deficiency. The hormone has the characteristic to minimize and regulate our appetite.

Serotonin and melatonin are a perfectly matched team in our body, which maintains the communication between our organs and thus influences our life expectancy and our efficiency. They should not be substituted by artificial hormones because there is a risk that our body will reduce or stop the production. Melatonin is the strongest antioxidants fighting free radicals.

We should not face any worries concerning cholesterol levels, moods and life expectancy if our body is sufficiently supplied with melatonin. Sadly, our modern life style does not always cater for an adequate supply of antioxidants like melatonin due to stress, bad lighting and environmental impacts. This might lead to stress reactions and the results are well known.

Environmental impacts like electro-smog have a very negative impact on human's melatonin levels. Scientific studies could show electromagnetic fields decrease the melatonin levels in humans. The people concerned used heating blankets or heating cushions, worked in laboratories or went through medical diagnostic methods.[48]

Our digital era marked by mobile phones and wireless LAN seems to have a particular reaction on the pineal gland and therefore the melatonin. The pineal gland, which is aligned on the Earths' magnetism is influenced by the modern devices and lowers the production of melatonin as a reaction. Diseases like cancer, leukemia, Alzheimer´s and depression are being discussed in this context.

In order to prevent a deficiency of melatonin we should spend sufficient time in the light of the sun, we should enjoy sunrises and sunsets and most importantly, allow for a natural rhythm.

Humans would like to control the entire universe but they keep forgetting we are only one part of the whole. One day hopefully, we will come to our senses and we will be able to live our life in our rhythm again.

Please note: Chronobiology = the doctrine of the rhythm in the organism (bio-rhythm)

- Parts of it are the sleep-wake cycle, jetlag, seasons and the phase of the moon etc.
- Sunlight is the most important timer for our bio-

rhythm
- The production of serotonin-melatonin, which is linked to sunlight, is very important for a healthy life, our sleep-wake rhythm, as well as, our life expectancy. Modern ways of living in artificial light, electro smog do very often and in many places not cater for a sufficient supply

D) Photosynthesis and Chlorophyll

Photosynthesis

We have all heard about photosynthesis during our days at school. This term is so common for most people they have started to forget the importance of the process. Our whole life depends on this bio-geo-chemical process of the Earth. It is one of the oldest biochemical processes of our planet and is activated by the sun. Geologists have found proof that the photosynthesis has been present for 3.5 to 4 billion years.

Without this process, there would be no life at all on Earth. Food, oxygen, building materials and energy are extracted from that process and CO_2 is broken down. Our green plants and some microorganisms, which have the ability to integrate sun energy into the circulation of nature, accomplish this miracle on a daily basis. During a complex procedure with the help of sunlight and their blood pigments made up of mainly the green chlorophylls, these creatures manage to break down water into its elements oxygen and hydrogen.

Photosynthesis activates all biochemical circulations in every ecological system on planet Earth. Under the current circumstances of solar energy radiation photosynthesis produces about 10^{11} tons of dry mass annually. Tropical rainforests are the main drivers of this production.

Photosynthesis does thus have several important factors because all green plants produce biomass and oxygen from water and air with assistance of sunlight. Carbon dioxide is extracted from the air for the process of the photosynthesis. At this point, the so-called carbohydrates are built by adding light radiation. This way, plants can grow and produce oxygen at the same time.

Plants, which have more access to sunlight, break down more CO_2 in comparison to plants that are positioned in the shade.

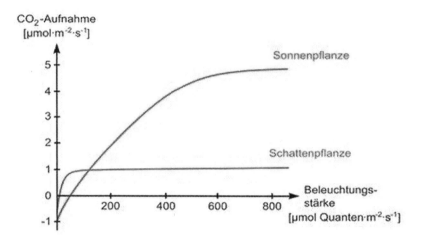

Correlation of photosynthesis rate (ordinate) to the available amount of light (abscissa) in sun – and shade plants[49] (red=sun plant="Sonnenpflanze", green=shade plant="Schattenpflanze")

One of life's important rules is we first have to breathe before we can eat and drink. Photosynthesis and respiration are proportional. By looking at the widely discussed change in climate, the answer concerning elevated CO_2 levels seems very simple. Stop cutting down the rain forests because we need many more trees and plants to absorb and process the CO_2. Additional information is provided in the chapter "sun activity and climate change".

A field related journal "Science" published an interesting report at the end of October 2011 stating that US scientists have managed to build a photosynthesis machine. The lightweight devise manages to convert sunlight into storable energy. The artificial leaf has the feature of being able to separate water, which is exposed to sunlight, into oxygen and hydrogen.

Well, we remember now that photosynthesis reduces carbon dioxide into rich energy compounds and therefore produces important energies for the bio-system of the Earth.

Chlorophyll

Decisive molecules in the photosynthesis apparatus of plants, algae and defined bacteria are the chlorophylls, which we need to consider further.

Chlorophyll is a Greek term and its meaning in English is "leaf green". And that is exactly what it is, the stuff, which allows the leaves to look green. We know already from the chapter on photosynthesis that plants produce carbohydrates from water and carbon dioxide (CO_2). They need a lot of energy for that process to work, which they draw from the sun.

The leaf green chlorophyll absorbs the light and thus enables the plant to produce building material. One of the characteristics is that chlorophylls like to cover a maximum area per plant in order to obtain optimal sunlight. That is why nature has furnished most plants with flat and green leaves.

However, what happens during autumn when the leaves become colorful in the northern hemisphere from Japan to Russia and Canada and not to forget Europe? The answer is easy; the inner clock of the plants realizes that there are less hours of sunlight and therefore the chlorophyll production is reduced to the point at which the tree will have lost all of its leaves in late autumn. This procedure is a self-protection mechanism of the plant. We have already heard a lot of this issue in the chapter on chronobiology.

Chlorophyll produces glucose from light and water, which feeds the trees. Every autumn, the trees extract energy from the leaves in order to deposit it into the stem. This natural procedure is very important for deciduous trees to ensure their survival because their water supply is regulated through the leaves. If there were still leaves left on the tree in winter, it would lose the important moisture at a difficult time of ground frost when it is already difficult to extract water. Of course there are exceptions, as the evergreen plants, which have the diverse characteristic to use only little water and food. It is different in cone trees because of their special characteristic that allows them to close their needles.

There are micro processes happening which we are hardly aware of. If our plants achieve such tremendous accomplishments by reacting very sensitively to the time of radiation and if in only a few minutes each day they manage to trigger enormous procedures, it is potentially easy to imagine what unforeseen powers are activated in humans by the sun. The sun has an important impact on our entire psychological and physical performance and therefore our wellbeing and I feel it is time to pay more attention to that issue.

Chlorophyll is very important in treatment prescribed by naturopaths because green foods add to vitality, accelerate the healing process and improve the total health scope. Chlorophyll supports detoxification in our bodies and assists the production of blood cells. Edible plants highly enriched with chlorophyll are vegetables, sprouts, herbs, and algae to name just a few. The formula of naturopathy is simple. It is the amount of chlorophyll in chlorophyll-rich food directly linked to the level of your potential health benefits?

Many naturopaths prescribe chlorophyll if the patient suffers from low iron , magnesium levels or from constipation; it also supports the natural wound healing. Due to detox procedures in our bodies, such as the one happening in the liver, we can obtain a pleasant body odor and could possibly do away with deodorants in future. Furthermore, the acid-base balance in the body will be recovered which has a regenerating and healing effect. The oxygen level in our body will increase as will our energy, our vitality and our performance power. As a result, our concentration and fitness will improve. The blood pressure is regulated and you will feel many years younger. Chlorophyll enables the metabolism of fat, strengthens and firms up the connective tissue removing cellulite. The listing of positive effects is very long and I could not find any negative characteristics of chlorophyll in the course of my research.

An article called "Chlorophyll the wonder of nature" was published online on May 19, 2010 starting with an impressive quotation by Ann Wigmore: "In the coming Age of Enlightenment the chlorophyll will be the main protein. It contains synthesized sunshine in every freshly prepared drink and the electric power, which is needed for the reactivation of the body, and it will make regions of our brain accessible of which humans do not know at present."[50]

The green juices are particularly popular in this context. Wheat grass juice and barley grass drinks are well known for their positive effects when it comes to high blood pressure, which is often caused by cholesterol and the narrowing of the blood vessels. If your were suffering from high cholesterol levels, the antioxidants 2-0-GIV would come into effect and might lower cholesterol levels as well as prevent the blood clotting. It means that the green power can be used for the prevention or healing of heart diseases. In Japan, barley grass extract contains a substance called beta levels.[51]

The benefits of green foods are indispensable for leading a healthy life.

The industrialization as well as our modern ways of living has regrettably brought drastic cuts. The responsibility of handling our nutrition is in our power because it is about our health. Therefore, we should not do without the green power foods. The following template shows a selection of vegetables and their chlorophyll content.[52]

Chlorophyll content in selected raw vegetables

Food	Serving	Chlorophyll (mg)
Spinach	1 cup	23.7
Parsley	½ cup	19.0
Garden cress	1 cup	15.6
Green beans	1 cup	8.3
Rocket	1 cup	8.2
Leek	1 cup	7.7
Endive	1 cup	5.2
Sugar pea	1 cup	4.8
Bok Choy Celery Cabbage	1 cup	4.1

All selected vegetables were tested as raw vegetables and should be eaten or drunk as such.

I have come across an interesting recipe by an Australian naturopath for a highly dosed vegetable juice some months ago. The ingredients are: 2 green peppers, 5 green apples, some red cabbage, 1 endive, 1 bunch of watercress, 1 bunch of green carrot leaves and some cos lettuce leaves also called roman salad. Wash all ingredients, put them into the juicer and enjoy the freshly pressed drink. Try it and see if you feel some changes; you might be more active, the liver is cleansed, scentless or you might have an efficient digestive tract and feel a lot younger.

On August 19, 2010 The Science Online Magazine published an article reporting about the discovery of a new chlorophyll molecule. The particular chlorophyll molecule has the characteristic of being able to absorb long-wave light within the near infrared limit.

The question asked by scientists was how plants with less sun exposure, due to them being hidden underneath larger leaves of other plants, still manage to produce chlorophyll. They observed this on Australian algae mats, the so called stromatolites, which belong to the oldest biological structures known on Earth. The upper layers of these algae mats had a much higher chance of light exposure compared to the lower layers. An international team of scientists led by the Australian botanist Prof. Min Chen reports: "We managed to show that the molecule was in its structure very similar to the `chlorophyll a´ but it could absorb much deeper within the infrared limits compared to the other four known chlorophylls."

The newly discovered chlorophyll is named `chlorophyll f´, which is the first new chlorophyll of oxygenic photosynthesis found in more than 60 years.

But what does the great discovery hold for us? One of the participating scientists Prof. Hugo Scheer biologist at the LMU explains it: "Technical equipment which operates with light as an energy source could gain a higher degree of efficiency by using these principles.

However, there are also medical methods. During the photodynamic therapy of cancer, light sensitive medication is collected in the tumor. They are activated by aiming light radiation from outside. In this context the chlorophylls, which absorb in the near infrared region are very interesting because the radiation within that spectral range can deeply penetrate into the tissue."[53]

The German chemist Richard Willstätter, who received the Nobel Prize of chemistry in 1915 for the isolation of the green color in plants (namely the chlorophyll), had already discovered it consisted of a combination of two chlorophylls – the blue-green `chlorophyll a´ and the yellow-green `chlorophyll b´.

Chemically, they are both related to the red blood pigment

`hemin´. Part of both chlorophylls is the pyrrol, which is an element of the blood pigment. The compound of hemin together with the protein globin forms the hemoglobin of our red blood cells. Through these, oxygen is transported into our tissue and energy and life becomes possible. We all depend on that cycle, which has its beginning in the light of our sun.

"Foils become yellow,

but every

year the book of nature receives a new issue."

(Hans Christian Anderson)

It is also called wonder of nature. It is a wonder, which would be impossible without the sun.

The yogis discovered these secrets and wonders of the sun as well.

E) Sun Meditation in Yoga

Let us take a break after all that science and let's have a look at our sun from a more relaxing perspective. It is the meaning of our sun in yoga. The healing and energizing effect of our sun is well known to the yogis. Historical traditions show that first rituals were practiced more than 5,000 years ago. It would take an additional book to explain all the varieties of yoga. At this point, we will concentrate on the aspect of the `Sun Salutes´, the so-called `Suray Namaskar´ in German `Sonnengruß´. An Australian yoga teacher who teaches at the Hinterland of the Sunshine Coast in Queensland, explains the pieces of wisdom to her students in the following way:

Sun Salutes is a sequence of 12 flowing movements, which symbolically relate to the sun as a representation of the essence of the universe. The sun revitalizes and promotes growth on Earth. It is also seen as a manifestation of the invisible, spiritual, inner light. Traditionally, Hatha yoga practice begins with a sequence of sun salutations, ideally facing east towards the sun. This warms up the body and energizes it, as well as awakening the breathing and bringing the mind into focus.

Each salutation begins and ends with the hands in the prayer position. Some call it the Namaste mudra. Namaste means: "I honor the place in you, in which the entire universe dwells - the place in you which is of love, light, peace and joy. When you are in that place in you and I am in that place in me – we are one! "

In ancient India, the yogis lived close to nature, experiencing deep communion with the elements of the sun, wind, fire, water, earth and ether. Saluting the sun was a ritual act of venerating life and creation.

In India, the number 108 is sacred, suggesting completeness and wholeness. It is widely used in different contexts. Scientists can see a connection between the Earth and the sun because the Earth will fit about 108 times into the diameter of the sun. The Hindu – and Buddhist rosary contains 108 pearls.

The advantage of facing the sun during the first half an hour of daylight is the special stimulating effect. Sunset is a good time to practice the sun salutes as it stimulates the digestive fire. Traditionally – surya namaskar is practiced in 9 sets of 12, which leads us back to the holy figure 108. Please see the 12 postures of the sun salutes, which should be repeated 9 times, as already explained.

Practice of Sun Salutes (Surya Namaste) German "Sonnengruß"

Yoga Sun Salute[54]

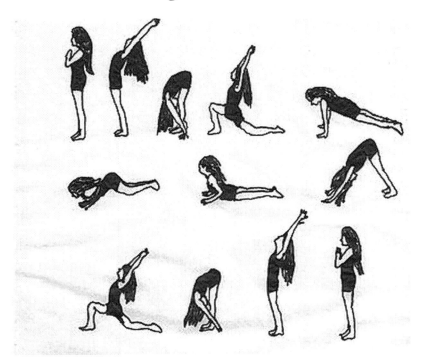

And what benefits can we draw from these exercises:

- Strengthens and increases flexibility throughout the entire body
- Improves circulation and the functioning of the immune system
- Improves breathing and the release of toxins through the breath and pores of the skin
- Tones the nervous system
- Improves digestion, assimilation, and elimination through a squeeze and soak massage of internal organs
- Removes lethargy and fatigue
- Develops a sense of mediation in movement integrating and harmonizing body and mind

- Develops an awareness of internal energy
- Stimulates all the chakras

**Caution:** Consult your health care provider if you suffer from high blood pressure, spinal or knee injuries.

Yogis have trusted in the strengthening power of the sun for many millennia. Perhaps, we should trust a little more, in particular the population of Western societies, in their fine traditional wisdom.

After the relaxing excursus, let us return to our everyday life namely the scientific forms of energy.

Please note:

1. The revitalizing power of our sun has been known by yogis for over 5.000 years
2. They honor the sun until today with the exercise of the sun salutes

6. Energy

A) Energy Saving Light per Ordinance

Sunlight and Artificial Lighting

Many states put the final nail in the coffin when they spelled the end of the traditional light bulb. Politics advertise the prospect of immense energy savings with the adoption of low-energy light bulbs. They also tell us that we save on CO_2 output. Countries and communities like the EU the United Nations, Switzerland, Cuba and others share this point of view.

Yet, what is the reality? Are the mathematical examples of our governments correct, does our choice in light bulbs really have an impact on the climate – or is the state ordinance on lighting very risky?

In order to get out of the dark, we should know some basics about the light being made available to us. Let's get started with the most natural form of light, namely our sunlight. The solar radiation is an electromagnetic radiation, which is spread over a wide spectral range. The spectral regions range from long radio waves to ultra-short X-rays. The radiation spectrum is roughly divided into radio waves, terra waves, infrared radiation, visible light, UV-radiation, X-rays, gamma rays and hard cosmic radiation. The visible solar radiation is only a small part in the total spectrum of our sun. The wavelength range of this radiation is measured in nanometers (nm), where one meter equals 1,000,000,000 nm, in other words, a very small unit of length. The wave length, which is visible for us humans, ranges from deep red (780nm) to ultra-violet (380nm). The energy of light particles (photons) generally increases with decreasing wavelength. In this context, we should not confuse radiation energy with radiation intensity because the energy is responsible for the energetic effect, the intensity stands for the radiation mass. In photochemical reactions, break molecular connections and new molecules evolve. In order to get this process of change started, it is important for the wavelength not to exceed a particular value. The energy of the radiation would be too little in a higher wavelength for this process, irrespectively of the extent of the intensity. The UV radiation, which adjoins the visual light, always has wavelengths, which become shorter and therefore have an increasing energy impact, which is of great importance to us.

The scope of UV-A and UV-B radiation hold enough radiation energy to trigger numerous photochemical processes in our body, likewise the synthesis of vitamin D 3.

One should be very cautious when it comes to UV-B and UV-C radiation (mainly from artificial light sources) and of course any other radiation with even shorter wavelengths because due to the very high energy other organic molecules can be literally demolished. That is also, why our body has natural repair mechanisms in our cells. However, if we expose ourselves for too long to the intense radiation or the energy rich radiation, our body will no longer be able to regenerate itself and early lasting damage to our skin (it will age quickly) and skin cancer will occur.

The Earth's atmosphere is, for the majority of the spectrum, impenetrable and therefore inaccessible or only accessible for these parts in a very limited form. That important characteristic of the Earth's atmosphere protects us as well from energy rich radiation. There would be no life on planet Earth without that important function.

However, life could only evolve with the presence of sunlight. Therefore, it has an important influence on the regulation and perpetuation of our life processes as well as our health and our well-being.

The natural day light condition varies in conjunction with the time of the day, the seasons, and the weather and of course the geographic location. Our bodies developed under various light conditions and thus produced suitable mechanisms to control and adjust the body functions and our visual perception.

Sunlight is a source of energy and information at once. The infrared radiation produces heat effects whilst the shorter wave lengths, in particular the UV-A and UV-B (up to 300nm), are important for photochemical processes. The visual light gives us exact information about our surroundings, which we perceive via the eye. At the same time it provides us with important information concerning the control of our bio rhythm as well as the day-night-rhythm (please see chapter chronobiology).

Vision is probably the most important one of our senses. The eye and the processing of visual impressions in our brain are highly complex. About 85 percent of all sensory perceptions are of a visual nature. Only about 20 percent of the light perceived by our eye is utilized for visualization the remaining ca. 80 percent are used to control biological functions. At this point, you might be able to assume the importance of good lighting.

The spectrum of penetrated light is dependent on two factors, namely from the spectral distribution of the lighting source and from the reflection characteristics of the lit objects. Only a portion of the light that shines onto the object is reflected, the other portion will be absorbed. The light, which falls into our eye, is a product mix between lighting and reflection and these two elements can therefore not be diverted at a later stage. You can quickly test this yourself. A green color impression can equally occur by lighting a white area with green lighting or by lighting a green area with white light.

However, our visual apparatus is by many means more evolved than mathematics. Mathematically, both examples lead to the same distribution of the wavelength. However, our visual system can still draw conclusions from the spectral reflection characteristics of the objects. We call this amazing procedure "color constancy". The color constancy makes use of the characteristic that the reflectance of objects is constant. We can notice this during the day when the light conditions change but the color impressions on objects remain. Yet, this also means that color does not have equal wavelength. Single colored light triggers under neutral circumstances always the same color sensation but vice versa, it is not possible to relate a particular wavelength to a particular color sensation. Natural objects in our surroundings always reflect light over a wide range of wavelengths and finally determine which color we see.

Furthermore, it is known we have more light sensitive sensors besides the cones and rods in the retina of our eye, which do not cater for vision but for sending optical impulses to the hypothalamus and from there into the pineal gland and pituitary gland. The hypothalamus is the central corridor of power from where vegetative nerve impulses and hormone signals evolve. The pituitary is responsible for the hormones and hangs as the pituitary gland on the hypothalamus.

The hypothalamus controls and regulates most of our life-sustaining functions, triggers and coordinates the reactions of stress influences and steers the pituitary, which regulates the endocrine system of the hormone producing glands (pineal gland, thyroid, parathyroid, thymus, adrenal glands, pancreas and gonad).

The pituitary does not only produce hormones, it also stores hormones being produced by the hypothalamus and releases them when necessary. Its activity is stimulated or restrained by the hypothalamus and by the hormones, which are produced by the glands. This reflection is important for our hormone balance. The pituitary regulates hormones like the growth hormones, stress hormones, thyroid hormones, sexual hormones, hormones that regulate the water balance, blood pressure, body temperature, the immune system etc. Can the serotonin – melatonin production be found in the same context? Please see the chapter concerning chronobiology.

Dr. Jacob Libermann explains in a very detailed way the various impacts on light regarding our life processes in his book "Light: Medicine of the Future". Today, it is assumed that different colors have differentiated impacts on the endocrine gland system and stimulate or restrain the hormone production in this way. Dr. Libermann relates to studies, which prove the influence of color on the sympathetic and parasympathetic nerve system, blood pressure, heart rate, respiration rate, migraines and physical exercise performance but also the effect of UV-light on our immune system.

Dr. John Nash Ott is a well-known pioneer in the science of the exposure to light on various forms of life. He believes the entire natural light spectrum is necessary to sustain a healthy life. He reports that light deficiency is a similarly colossal problem for the Western World, just like malnutrition. In his opinion, depression, a state of exhaustion, strained eyes, headaches, stress and illness can all be attributed to bad lighting. Above all, he has accumulated considerable data connecting the lack of sunlight and use of artificial lights with major diseases such as cancer and arthritis. He has managed to show the use of full spectrum light for schoolchildren, which was close to daylight, improved the scholar's concentration and calmed them. This way, he demonstrated the impact of various light sources on the hormone system, which influences the body and psyche.[55]

Prof. Fritz Hollwich, who has been working in the field of Ophthalmology in Germany for many years, specializes very intensively on the visual and energetic functions of the sight apparatus. He too has managed to prove studies the high importance of light on our health, well-being and regulating effects of the body in several. In one of his studies, he directly managed to show the dangerous influence of bad artificial light: Individuals sitting under cool white fluorescent tubes had high levels of stress hormones – specifically, the adrenocorticotrophic hormone (ACTH) and cortisol. However, people working under full spectrum tubes had normal levels.[56]

Many impacts of light on our bodies have not been fully researched but they are more and more moving into the spotlight of science.

The ordinance of energy saving lights by our governments and the ban of the traditional light bulb have provoked serious controversial discussions.

Official quarters tell us the light quality of energy saving lights is almost adequate compared to the light bulbs but they have the advantage of enormous energy savings.

The quality of light concerning lighting functions is calculated for us on the grounds of color temperature and color index (Ri). However, are these calculations really correct?

The energy saving type of light, which is offered to us as an alternative to the good old-fashioned light bulb is the compact fluorescent light and increasingly LED lighting. However, if you compare the spectrum of these types of lighting with the one of our daylight, it is immediately obvious that daylight does not exist in such a spectral distribution, not even remotely. Therefore, the light offered to us is unnatural light. Only portions of the full light spectrum are particularly present in compact fluorescent lights and some are missing completely. However, the light of the traditional bulb lighting is, in contrast, very similar to day light; its spectrum is continuous and consists of all shades of color. The daylight during sunset complies very much with the light of a halogen bulb lamp. The spectrum of an ordinary light bulb is even redder and has therefore a warmer color shade. Both light bulbs create in us the sensation of a late afternoon sun. This suits our needs of nature. How is it possible for the producers of the new light to cheat on these facts? The trick is easy because light in lighting technology is defined and marketed by the color temperature. But what does the color temperature tell us? In order to understand this, we should look at some fundamental principles. We should start with the definition of color temperature.

The color impression caused by a self-luminous body (the perceived light color) can be measured by the color temperature (stated in Kelvin). The perception of the color temperature is ideally recorded by comparing a black body. Is that body heated, it will release electromagnetic radiation. Alternatively, to put it more simply, just imagine you were at a blacksmith's, who is heating the material. Depending on the temperature, the material will have a different color. As the temperature increases, the color will change from a dark red to light red, white and finally into a bluish white. Each color is correlated with a temperature during the heating process, which is called color temperature. If we held our lightings (light bulb, fluorescent light) next to the heated material, the color temperature of the lighting would be the one, at which the color of the heated material and the lighting would match (heat measured in Kelvin). For professional measurements, of course, you would not go to the blacksmith. A specially produced black body is used for this purpose. The color temperature is the value, which correlates to the temperature to which the black body has to be heated in order to gain a matching light impression to the comparing light source as described more simply before. This is a very easy way of comparing light sources in regards to their color effect.

However, this method is massively disadvantaged, the light temperature does not reflect on the composition of the light spectrum and therefore does not say much about the color reproduction quality in rooms, which are lit by these light sources. This means in layman terms a compact fluorescent light and a light bulb with the same color temperature do not have the same quality in color rendering. Rooms, which are lit with light of the same light color, have different effects on us because of the differences in the spectral composition of the lights.

In order to eliminate this disadvantage, some of the producers additionally print the color-rendering index (Ra) next to the color temperature onto the packages of energy saving lights. This means, we can choose the quality of the color rendering in addition to the light color.

Yet color rendering, again, to me sounds to me like gobbledygook. During the old times with traditional light bulbs, the consumer was not bothered and confused with any of these terms!

If the color-rendering index has a data of 100 it means an optimal color rendering, which is at its best. Traditional light bulbs as well as halogen bulb lamps have almost always a Ra of 100 and offer therefore the best color rendering – there is no need to print it onto the packaging. The compact fluorescent lights are always worse, due to their principle of their color rendering as light bulbs. LED lighting is also not able to hold a candle up to the light bulb.

Therefore the color rendering index informs us to what extend the color rendering of an energy saving light is worth in comparison with the light of a traditional light bulb.

However, is it really guaranteed that a high Ra index like 90 has more or less the same color rendering quality as a light bulb? These false believes can quickly lead to a fatal disappointment.

The Ra data is determined by a standardized technique, which uses the color rendering of 8 pastel colors. This does not include tests on the color rendering quality of saturated colors meaning obtrusive, bright and conspicuous colors are not being tested. We perceive our surroundings in a great color variety, which cannot be reduced to just a few pastel colors. If we prefer bright and conspicuous colors in our environment it might be that we perceive those colors suddenly as matt and different in the light of compact fluorescent lighting. The color of a bright, conspicuous yellow blouse might appear as matt and green-yellow unless viewed in a, in comparison, good light of a light bulb. That is the crux of the matter. Industry chooses a method to determine the light rendering quality of their products only on the basis of 8 test colors. Strictly speaking, the Ra data accounts only to those 8 colors. None of this would be a problem regarding light bulbs, as their spectral progression is very similar to the ones of natural light conditions. If there is a distinct variation of the spectral light distribution and natural light (likewise in compact fluorescent lights), the Ra is no longer independent of the testing conditions and therefore no longer generally acceptable. If different test colors were chosen like saturated color tones, the Ra data would be different and could perhaps be worse. Therefore, the lighting industry optimizes their fluorescent lights to the color rendering of the test colors.

What does that mean to us if we have high requirements of color-rendering? We can only use the industries test colors when choosing light even if the Ra data needs to match our requirements. For consumers who do not like this arrangement, it is best to stick to the halogen bulb lamp or test the color impact of diverse energy saving lights. There are huge differences in quality regarding the products on offer.

In your living area, a color temperature for a warm-white light in the range of 2700K to 3200K is recommended. Generally, LED lighting should be preferred, as it does not contain the highly dangerous mercury. It has a continuously light spectrum, which is however not very well balanced.

Here is a short summary for the consumers. The color-rendering of compact fluorescent light and fluorescent tubes is marked with an international light color number. For example, an energy saving lamp with the identification "827" is extra warm-white. The first number identifies the color-rendering level, which is determined by the color-rendering index Ra:

4 = color-rendering level 1B (Ra 40 – 49)
5 = color-rendering level 1B (Ra 50 – 59)
6 = color-rendering level 1B (Ra 60 – 69)
7 = color-rendering level 1B (Ra 70 – 79)
8 = color-rendering level 1B (Ra 80 – 89)
9 = color-rendering level 1A (Ra ≥ 90)

The second and third number identifies the color temperature in Kelvin:

827 = extra warm-white 2700 K
830 = warm-white 3000 K
840 = neutral-white 4000 K
860 = daylight-white 6000 K [57]

Castigators argue in controversial discussions that compact fluorescent lights often flicker and therefore impact on our well-being.

Experts argue that modern compact fluorescent lights are equipped with electronic ballasts and that the flickering is therefore rendered unimportant.

This is false!

The luminous flux vibrates not only with the high switching frequency but also with the 100Hz half-wave frequency of the lighting main. The level of distinction regarding this effect depends on the quality (smoothing characteristics of the ballast) and the inertia of the used fluorescent substances.

There are substantial differences in quality but the consumers are being kept in the dark. The author had some compact fluorescent lights of the type GENIE, Cool Daylight, 18W from Phillips tested and they resulted to a "proud" value of 45 %. This means that the lamp divides its brightness 100 times in one second almost in half. This should not be called unimportant. Such low frequent light signals impact on our brain flow. It does not matter whether we are aware of these sensations or not. Either way, they have a negative impact on neurological processes, hormone balance, metabolism, nervousness and may cause headaches and migraines.

Natural light does not know such constant flickering. Due to their quick switching behavior fluctuations of up to 100 % in light luminance might occur. This depends on the ballast in individual cases. Most ballast are equipped with producing an intermittent direct current, meaning the LED will be switched on and off for about 40.000 times per second with the switching frequency of the ballast. However, the high frequency cannot be perceived due to the persistence of vision. There are no systematical studies concerning possible unconscious effects. If you changed, your lighting and you suddenly suffer from unexplained migraine headaches or indisposition it is possible that you are exposed to a high luminous ripple, which is responsible for the problems.

To put an end onto the traditional light bulb was a very unconsidered and imbalanced act. The matter should not rest there. Meanwhile, numerous doctors and scientist warn about the many risks to general health. They blame several illnesses on the bad lighting. Since the very beginning of humankind, our organisms and therefore our hormone balance are harmonized with the natural light of the sun during the day and flames during darkness. The regular and harmonic light spectrum of both natural light sources can be observed in a spectroscope. Sunlight has, compared to the flame, a higher blue purity, which changes closer to sun set into red. The flame with its high red purity mediates this sensation. The glowing tungsten wire in traditional light bulbs mediates exactly that feeling – the sensation of the late afternoon sun.

This is different in energy saving lamps. They consist of a much higher blue purity. In other words, they mediate the impression during the evening that it is day. This leads to a change in our hormone balance because the wrong signal is perceived. Therefore, our melatonin production does not adapt to the daytime but it orientates itself instead on the artificial light resulting in a stress reaction. In this context, health professionals mention sleeping disorders as well as a higher risk for developing diabetes, osteoporosis, cardiovascular diseases, and an increased risk for developing cancer as well as eye diseases.

Dr. Alexander Wunsch, a doctor based in Heidelberg, Germany, specializes in the therapeutic use of light and light biology. "Oeko Test" a German consumer magazine interviewed him concerning possible health risks and he explained the following:

"A distribution of high blue purity as found in energy saving lamps can cause false hormonal reactions, which over time promote (middle- and long term) the development of several lifestyle disorders like cardiovascular diseases. The body adapts to conditions, which do not really occur. Furthermore, bright bluish light activates the pituitary gland and then produces light stress. Further toxic effects can be observed in the eye. Blue light can pass the cornea and eye lens and penetrates fully into the retina. Experiments on cells have proven that it is possible for that type of light to harm the retina. Furthermore, many studies show that too much light at nighttime prevents the production of melatonin and encourages breast cancer in women. The blue purity of the artificial lighting is responsible for this. The diseases are not only triggered by those circumstances, other risk factors have to be present as well."[58]

Other health professionals like Dr. Colin Holden, president of the British Association of Dermatologists (BAD) reported as early as January 2008 in the Daily Mail, "It is important that patients who suffer from abnormal photosensitive skin sensitivity are allowed to use a lighting that does not worsen their condition ..."[59]

To summarize, it can be concluded the right light at the right time of the day plays a consequential important role for our well-being.

Could it be ambitious manufacturers and members of parliament have overlooked the health aspects because all they looked at was the savings?

It is a fact that light interferes in all biological life proceedings thus controlling the hormone balance and cell metabolism. The absorption of light is processed via the skin and our eyes. From there energy impulses will be transferred to the brain, which has an influence on the hypothalamus and pituitary as well as others. The hypothalamus controls reactions like breathing, blood pressure and our sleep-wake cycle. The pituitary interferes in a regulatory manner with the metabolism and the release of hormones of further glands. The type of lighting offered to us should not be treated as a second rate issue.

Politics beg to differ!

Americas advertising campaign runs as follows – if every household was to exchange one light bulb with a lighting carrying the "Energy Star", enough power would be saved to provide electricity for 3 million homes for a whole year. This equalizes the pollution emissions of 800.000 vehicles per annum.[60]

Germany wants to save so much the savings will equate to the closure of a nuclear power station.

The German Electrical and Electronic Manufacturers Association (Zentralverband Elektrotechnik- und Elektronikindustrie – ZVEI) announced that due to the EU-consent up to 4.5 million tons of climate-damaging carbon dioxide could be saved and that private households could be credited in the amount of 1.3 billion Euros.

All of those arguments are very interesting because none of them provide any information about the genuine influences, which the savings really have on our climate. Of course, these figures seem impressive and monumental but how could they be seen and understood realistically?

In order to answer this question it is important to consider the total emissions of carbon dioxide. This total was, according to the IPCC, 33.5 billion tons for the year 2010.

4.5 million tons in Germany in relation to the total of the emissions in 2010 are only 0.013 %. To date, no proof by any technique of measurement has been provided that even 100 % could have an important effect on our climate. Therefore, what effects would 0.013% or 0.1% or 1% have on savings?

To draw such comparisons can only serve propagandistic purposes and does not show any realistic relations. Nevertheless, they are necessary in order to understand the realistic impact.

As a method for a resolution, long lasting durable goods could be produced instead of useless junk. This could result in immense savings of raw materials and energy.

The formula seems clear as daylight for politics – the traditional light bulb wastes too much energy, which results in CO_2 emissions that are too high, which implies an avoidable greenhouse effect.

What impact can alleged 0.5 % savings have on our climate if the effect of the total emission cannot be proven by technical measurement methods and as the case may be, the effect has no real significance on our climate?

The experts in Brussels obviously use different mathematics. That is why they decided to gradually ban the light bulbs until the end of 2012.

In 2007, the USA decided in the Energy Independence and Security Act on the successive tightening of laws on the energy efficiency of light bulbs between the years 2012 and 2014. Irrespectively, of regulated exceptions like colored light bulbs, the traditional bulbs are banned by this act.[61]

New Zealand has an exemplarily different approach:

New Zealand decided against a ban. Over two decades ago, New Zealand already researched the way in which the consumption of electricity could be minimized. A research group of the University of Auckland published findings stating that 90 % of the total CO_2 emissions in New Zealand can be blamed on electric power consumption in the World Resource Review. Despite the difficulty regarding the sourcing of comparable figures it could be demonstrated that one of the Universities managed to minimize the power consumption from 219 kWh/m (2) Yr. in 1979 to 130 kWh/m (2) Yr. in 1994 by using their electricity consciously. For example, the heating temperature was reduced to an acceptable level and lights were switched off during times of sufficient day light. This amounted to a minimization in consumption of 20 to 50 percent.[62]

Despite being a pioneer in the matter of energy saving lamps New Zealand surprised the world when the Minister for Energy and Resources, Gerry Brownlee, announced in parliament on 16.12.2008 that the ban on traditional light bulbs would be being lifted. He said, "This government has real concerns about telling people they have to move to energy efficient light bulbs by decree." He further commented: "It has been well signaled and will come as no surprise the government is lifting the ban on traditional or incandescent light bulbs. We are committed to energy efficiency in the home and efficient lighting has an important role to play in helping us reduce the amount of energy we use, but this Government believes it is a matter of consumer choice. People need good, credible information about the different lighting options that are available to them, and then they can decide what is right for them in their homes. Lifting the previous government´s ban on incandescent light bulbs simply means we are allowing their continued sale, and I am confident the customer trend to energy efficient bulbs will continue."[63]

Yet, in Great Britain, as well the discussion concerning energy saving lights continues. More and more voices opposing the new energy saving lights are making themselves heard.

The trigger for these discussions is the damaging effects these light providers supported by political propaganda have on human health.

Mercury, electro smog as well as light quality are classified as potential health risks. The decreed light only functions by utilizing the highly toxic heavy metal mercury.

The compact fluorescent lamps contain mercury that evaporates at room temperature. The mercury vapor is forced to glow by high voltage. In order to evaporate the entire mercury present in the lamp, the mercury is heated. The spectrum of the mercury light is not continuous; it contains rather intensive lines within the visible range at 577nm, 546nm, 436nm and 405nm as well as many spectral components within the UV range, whereby the strongest line can be found at 365nm. This light activates the light producing substances in the glass bulb, which in turn produce light. This means that the light of a fluorescent lamp does not only consist of activated fluorescent substances but also of the glowing mercury vapor spectrum.

Some years ago, The German Federal Environment Agency (Umweltbundesamt – UBA) criticized the energy saving lamps for their mercury content. Nevertheless, the levels are not supposed to be dangerous. It is said that the measured concentration is so small that it could be disregarded and it would not be harmful to health. However, meanwhile warnings have been published, which state it is necessary to ventilate a room in which an energy saving bulb burst for 15 minutes and the remains should be removed. Yet, it should not be cleaned with a vacuum cleaner because mercury could be spread.

The light bursting during operation is especially dangerous as it is hot. Due to the immediate cooling of the gaseous mercury, a large part condenses and contaminates therefore the entire room!!! It is then advisable to have the danger of the situation checked by an expert before serious damage is caused to someone's health. Ventilation does not make a huge difference in such a dangerous situation. Mercury stored in the body acts as a neurotoxin.

Meanwhile, the European Union restricted the mercury content with an EU Directive to five milligram per unit/lamp.

However, that too is no protection from health damages because as little as 5 mg can be sufficient to cause significant health risks. This always depends on circumstances.

In Germany, energy saving lights are treated as hazardous waste because of their toxic substances. The question is how many of those lamps do really end in hazardous waste sites. The shocking answer is less than a fifth.

The European Commission decreed as early as 2005 in a Mercury-Minimization-Program (Gemeinschaftsstrategie für Quecksilber 2005/2050 (INI)) that as from April 2009 no measurement instruments containing mercury, as e.g. thermometers, may be sold. Another UN-World program fights for the minimization of mercury in our environment. Yet, despite of all of that knowledge everybody in charge seems to backpedal when it comes to the compact fluorescent light.

An Australian Newspaper `Die Woche´ published on January 29, 2013 an article stating that 140 states managed to find a binding Convention according to international law concerning the reduction of toxic mercury. Achim Steiner the executive director of the UN-Environment Program explains this could reduce the health risk for millions of people on a global scale. He mentions furthermore the risks regarding mercury had been known for over a century. At the least 15 years after the commencement of the contract the production of mercury should widely be stopped. The contract is also called "Minamata Convention" because thousands of people suffered health damages and deadly diseases on the central nervous system in the 1950th due to mercury toxins that had gotten into the waterways. Mercury should not just be banned in most industrial practices but also in energy saving lamps, electrical circuits, cosmetics, thermometers and blood pressure monitors.[64] Meanwhile we continue to simply keep our eyes closed. Let us dive into some more controversies.

In April 2011, another study conducted by the German Television channel NDR a consumer and economy magazine called "Markt" saw the light of day. The study found that energy saving lights could cause cancer. The eco-lights release toxic substances like phenol into the environment. That though is not the tip of the iceberg because "Markt" commissioned tests, which could prove a veritable cocktail of toxic substances, which could pollute the indoor air.

The German Federal Environmental Agency arrived at a controversial result. On the April 21, 2011, they published a response concerning the alleged phenol – and aromatic vapors: "The concentration of volatile organic compounds from energy saving lights indoor is expected to be very small. There is no fear of health related impacts."[65]

The Swiss Federal Office for Health (Schweizer Bundesamt für Gesundheit – BAG) ordered another study concerning the electromagnetic fields of energy saving lights. The organization "Foundation for Research on Information Technologies in Society, Zurich", which conducted the research, introduced data in March 2010 stating that the levels of the tested energy saving lights stayed within international recommended norms.

Despite the findings that energy saving light is apparently harmless the Federal Agencies have recommend a safety distance to energy saving lights of at least 30 cm as a precautionary measure. This is particularly true, if the light is operated over a longer period, such as a desk lamp.[66] The study also checked on the electromagnetic fields of traditional light bulbs and LED lamps. Compared to the energy saving lamps, they produced only very weak electromagnetic fields.

Note on limits: A generalization there is no danger if levels go below a certain limit is wrong.

The limit itself, depending on time analysis and combinational interactions as well as individual conditions of the exposed person, should not be underestimated.

If all the limits protected us so well, then the epidemiology of the past 50 years would have been a very different one.

All the different norms, codes and certification directives within the EU are very confusing for consumers. For example, the Swedish TCO – seal for ergonomic quality regulates the certification of computer monitors within office environments.

Eco lamps exceed the levels considerably, which are set by the TCO certification for low radiation monitors at a distance of 30 cm.

A Swiss citizen organization called `Buergerwelle´ claims to know that a single energy saving lamp exudes 10 - to 40 times more emissions onto the head of the work place user during its operating frequency and at a distance of 30 cm as a modern monitor.[67] Therefore, energy savings lights are not suitable for work places.

The consumers are confused by all the tangled mass of all the studies and it becomes very difficult to make the right decisions.

It is unbelievable that studies like the one from the BAG in Switzerland state, on the one hand, the new light is harmless but, at the same time, warns of strong electromagnetic fields.

As early as November 1988, Osram promoted the compact fluorescent lamp with the heading: "The Bulb has Matured".

Maybe, the energy saving aspect is only half the truth, the other missing half might be the stimulation of the industries' sales.

Another very controversial issue is the aspect of how much energy is really saved by the new light.

The figures vary from the published figures of the Governments to only one percent savings capacity of the total energy consumption. Anyhow it can be verified that our climate is not tangent or only at a regardless small percentage – a percentage which is not scientifically proven.

Greenpeace got agitated over the ban of the climate killing lamps. Greenpeace supporter protested in many actions against the trade of traditional lighting. That is why they destroyed 10,000 traditional light bulbs with a road roller in front of the `Brandenburg Tor´ in Berlin in April 2007. The anti-light bulb action came with the slogan "Save the Climate". This slogan should be continued with - … and destroy our environment – because about 80 percent of the energy saving lights, which contain toxic mercury, ends up in our domestic waste. This way the groundwater can potentially be contaminated for generations to come.

The French Ministry for Ecology and Sustainable Development announced the following EU-goal in 2005. If the energy efficiency increases by 20 percent until the year 2020 – 1 million new jobs could be established in Europe. Today, the reality looks very different because the bulb manufactures have moved to China and the East.

Let us once more have a quick look at energy efficiency. It is correct that energy saving lights save electricity. The governments praised a saving of 80 percent; however, the study of Eco-Test draws a different picture. Eco-Test included the factor "brightness" into their testing because most energy saving lights are not as bright conventional ones and they tested a burning period of 2.000 hours.[68] The saving lights of Osram and General Electric showed good results whilst the majority showed a mere saving between 50 and 70 percent. Further disadvantages were present concerning the duration. The new lights are very sensitive if switched on and off frequently and they are not as durable as believed.

The new light seems much more dimmed and consumers tend to turn on more lights – without raising any objections to energy saving.

Psychological effects play a decisive role because many consumers think of it along the lines of "I am a climate protester by buying the new lights" and because of the peace of mind, the lights are kept on without wasting a further thought. Some consumers tend to increase the room temperature as well because warmth felt caused by the white light of the saving lamps is less. People miss in particular the warm color in the light; colors, like the natural ones being produced by our sun.

The light quality in particular is a cause of concern. It is said that the light color differs significantly from the one found in natural light. However, the color of traditional light bulbs is very similar to natural light. Furthermore, the energy saving lights flicker like a light storm in the perceivable range. Eco-Test blames headaches, dizziness, feeling unwell, neurological disorders and hormone problems on the bad light.[69]

The study of Eco-Test also proved the new lights are not as bright as the traditional light. This can be detected according to the manufacturer´s instructions. Luminous flux is measured in industrial standards in `Lumen´. The new light ranges between 347 and 660 Lumen. An old 60W light bulb measures 710 Lumen. Only very, few models of the new light have the same brightness as a 60W traditional light bulb. The review becomes even more drastic after a burning period of 2.000 hours. The new lights tend to lose their brightness over time. Precious light is also wasted during the warm up phase of the new lights, which might take up to five minutes.

Is it because of all these reasons that New Zealand's government opted against the ban of traditional light bulbs?

The new light has been discussed for over a decade but consequently, there are still no long-term studies regarding risks involved. It would have been wiser to collect sufficient evidence from responsible first, neutral and serious sources before implementing the new light.

Results retrieved with an open mind would have brought to light the pros and cons and consequently the consumers would have had a fair chance to form an ultimate opinion on energy savings coupled with all the risks involved.

Energy saving lights do save electricity but they do so on the account of our health and well-being! A better approach would have been to search for savings without incurring health risks.

Saving light is economically worthwhile in industrially lit rooms, which have to be kept cool and which are not often entered by people like storerooms, surfer rooms, archives etc. They might also be useful in places, where constant lighting is necessary but where there are not many people like in corridors and cellars. Savings could be accounted for if used outside, in driveways and streets – however, the effects on the surrounding fauna and flora needs to be taken into account.

Did you know the history of our street lighting is not very old, despite flambeaux? During the years between 1840 and 1850, the first forms of street lighting were introduced. Back then, the cloudy light was fed by rapeseed oil. In 1858, petroleum lamps replaced oil lamps. That type of lighting remained for many years until the gas light took over. After the invention of the Auer`schen mantle, the gas light was thought to be the best method of lighting. At the turn of the century (1900), many gas lamps were installed in larger cities. From 1850, various types of light bulbs were explored. Due to many legal disputes over patents, it is not possible to determine the exact origin. William David Coolidge a staff member of General Electric managed to develop a method for producing a mechanically stable tungsten filament in the year 1910. In 1911, General Electric started the mass production of light bulbs with a tungsten filament. They continued to be traded until our days. Furthermore, long life light bulbs with burning durations of more than 10,000 hours have been developed by smaller manufacturers. Yet, they were not to reach the consumer as the powerful manufacturers feared for their profits. This was just a very brief excursion into history.

Let us return to the energy saving lamps of our times:

The lights should be used with caution in living rooms, bedrooms and studies. They should be avoided in children's rooms.

"The Poem on the Bulb" sums it up:

The Poem on the Bulb

The economist in Brussels says tough:
"The old lamp is not good enough,
Because like every citizen here knows
the light is bright, the lamp's heat shows."
The economist conclusion is thus reached
too much electricity this lamp needs,
and because it has been preached for years
the households should save without fears.
Brussels got ready for action
to ban the lamp with high attraction.
And as a special gift in store
a substitute is found for all
the lamp sporting the nasty light
which doesn´t surprise me in the slight,
for a long time there's been a remark
in Brussels many things stay in the dark.
Now, to every citizen it's clear as day
why the old light couldn't stay.

(German version by Rajabeat, 26.3.2009)
(English version by Elisabeth J. Ellmer, 14.02.2013)

B) Solar Power

Most people think immediately about roofs covered with solar panels when hearing or reading the term solar power. Yet, solar energy means a lot more than that. The term "solar" stands for "concerning the sun" and means the energy, which the sun produces deeply within releasing it to the surface from where it is radiated. This solar energy is highly important to us because, as we have learned from previous chapter, no life would be possible on Earth without it. This form of energy is very interesting because it is available to us free of charge and seems to be unlimited. This enormous energy potential is responsible for many processes on the Earth's surface. Our climate and weather are also determined by the sun just like life, as discussed in the chapter on photosynthesis. This results in several forms of energy like wind power, geothermic, water power and bio energy.

However, the most commonly used form of sun power is that of photovoltaic. This process means no other than the transfer of sun energy, which appears in the form of radiations, into electrical energy, which we call solar power.

A study released by the market research company GTM Research (Cambridge, Massachusetts, USA) in 2011 shows Germany leads globally regarding photovoltaic (pv) installations with 7,4 GW in 2010. However, an article published on the 8th of February 2013 concerning predictions and prospects for the year 2013 forecast a third place for Germany behind China and the United States.[70]

Estimated global photovoltaic installations, 2010 (MW-dc)[71]

Germany	7,437
Italy	1,487
USA	910
Czech Republic	850
Rest of Europe	585
Japan	541
France	540
Spain	410
China	373
Canada	295

Rest of the world	209
South Korea	132
India	102
Rest of Asia	83
Greece	81

The calls for renewable energies got louder after the dramatic events following the tsunami in Japan early in 2011. China announced, for example, the doubling of its solar energy aims in the near future. The market research company GTM Research published a report in February 2011 stating the global photovoltaic materials will grow by 50 percent until the year 2014.[72]

The clean solar energy is available to an almost unlimited extent and no CO_2 emissions develop, only during the production of the panels. The only disadvantage is the waste disposal of the panels as they consist partly of polluting substances like silicon. On the other hand, people are more independent from fossil fuels like coal, gas and oil when using photovoltaic constructions. The total amount of energy released by the sun to Earth is many times higher than the energy need of today's civilization. It is estimated to be about 5,000 times higher. The largest disadvantage is the dependence on location. Countries, which are closer to the equator, have more sun. Countries and Continents, and States like Africa, the Middle East, Chile, Australia, California or India have many more hours of sun exposure than other regions on Earth. These countries naturally offer the best utilization. Countries like Germany are very dependent on weather conditions, seasons and therefore the solar altitude. Especially during the winter months, when more electricity is required, solar radiation is somewhat lacking. Then the days are short, the nights are long and storage is a problem. Due to the constant reduction of pay back rates to consumers, investments into solar power installations are no longer as profitable as during the early days of this industrial branch. Households are stuck with ever-increasing expenses for their electricity. In the beginning, expensive alternative developments of energy received high subsidizations such as wind energy and solar power. Meanwhile, they turned into shocking cost scenarios. Decisions concerning such forms of energy are mainly based on data provided by the Intergovernmental Panel on Climate Change (IPCC) on global warming. However, that seems far from the truth because the evidence and voices that global warming is not taking place are stacking up.

Well, systematically Australia as well is in the process of reducing the subsidies for solar power. The sunny state of Queensland for example produced so much energy the power lines are overloaded. As consumers are still entitled to receive their pay back rates by the government, it has worked to be an expensive exercise and huge burden on the state's budget.

The installations take up a lot of space and they are therefore not always profitable to install on every building. The investment expenditures are still very high. Another thing that has to be kept in mind is the discussion regarding the storage of solar energy. Several methods are being tested because if the sun is not shining this method of energy production quickly results in disadvantages. Storage methods for solar energy, which are in development, are the sol-zinc method and the electrolysis. The electrolysis resulted in the production of methanol, which can be stored in tanks. In this way, electric power can be produced with the assistance of a fuel cell at any time.

In Africa, storage is not too big a problem because metropolitan areas like Johannesburg in South Africa have over 300 sunny days on record annually. However, South Africa does still not produce sufficient energy supply like most African countries. One reason for this is that only a few families are wealthy enough in Africa to pay for the basic costs of solar installation. The other reason is many rural villages and farms are too far removed from power lines, which they could feed in order to receive paybacks by the governments. Escom a South African energy supplier has still not signed any consumer agreements concerning paybacks. In rural regions, where the installations would be needed most, there is only little or no information, money or technically educated staff. Until this can change in the wider future, women will continue to collect and carry a lot of fire wood to their homes on top of their heads in order to be able to do the cooking. For quite some time now, South Africa has had a shortage regarding its power supply. The governments of the past apartheid area missed the boat in regards to timely investment and installation of power lines. Here, solar energy would be a great source as there is plenty of sunshine.

However, the issue is a little trickier for African developing countries. Urgently needed electricity for clean drinking water and the improvement of hygienic and medical conditions can only be paid for with credit from Europe. If we further consider corruption in our calculations, the power received from the sun and many projects become quickly unattainable for these countries. Many African states are dependent on industrial nations and perhaps a new approach needs to be found.

In Europe, however, the first plans for harnessing the power from Africa are already in the pipeline. The European company consortium – Munich Re, Siemens, German Bank, RWE as well as eight other members of the DII (Desertec Industrial Initiative - aim to import 15 percent of the total European electricity demand from nine solar thermal plants in Africa via a gigantic cable network. The project in the planning is not about photovoltaic but about solar heat. This principle uses high boiling liquid in tubes, which is heated by the technique of reflectors. This produces water vapor via a heat exchanger, which activates the turbines for power production. However, there are many catches. First of all, the budget, the project is estimated at 400 billion Euros, a minimum of 30 high voltage power lines are necessary. Then, there are logistic difficulties between the concerned countries, the transmission loss over long distances as well as the political instability of some countries and the protection against violations by rebels. The German Newspaper "Handelsblatt" reported on October 25, 2011 the project is rapidly progressing and a mega solar plant is already planned for Morocco. The first electricity delivery is expected to materialize between 2014 and 2016. The energy will cater for Morocco and will be exported to Europe. It is planned the power from Africa shall cater for a sixth of Europe's electricity demand by 2050. The project is of great concern to consumers because it is owned by only a few large corporations, which like to push up the prices for the improvements paid for by the dependent consumers. You can all already feel them, the rapidly rising costs of energy. This technique of electricity supply raises great concerns when taking dangers into account like corporate greed, corruption and political banter. Is it not today's reality that large-scale consumers who waste huge amounts of power are entitled to receive heavy discounts from electricity manufacturers whilst the ordinary person on the street has to dig deeper into his pockets.

In this context, we should keep a close eye on the developments of "Geo-engineering", namely the large scale targeted technical intervention of humans on the climate. It aims to control sun radiation by means of modern technology in order to cool our planet Earth.

You can read more about this in the chapter of climate change. The efficiency of solar plants would be compromised by the implementation of such technologies. Should not the whole of humanity be entitled to affordable solar energy? The question of whether the renewable energies are inevitable for the global future is still undecided for many countries.

Perhaps human kind will manage to overcome technical and human obstacles like the greed for profit in order to profit from "free energy" for all of us.

The German Federal Ministry of Economy and Technology released the following figures in 2012:

Renewable Energies in Germany – in Petajoule[73]

	2000	2010	2011
Water-power	92	75	65
Wind-energy	35	136	176
Photovoltaic	0,3	42,1	69,6
Timber, straw other solid materials	210	532	491
Biodiesel other liquid fuels	13	191	183
Waste and landfill gas	39	106	109
Sewage gas incl. biogas	20	292	350
Others*	9	39	43
Total	417	1413	1486
Percentage end energy consumption	4,5	15,2	17,0

* Solar -, Geothermic and heat pumps

The whole world seems to participate in the race for the largest solar power plant. I tried to research which countries are leading the current statistics in regards to launching the largest plants. America and China are trying to become number one. Also, Australia has ambitions and great plans for the future. Up to the beginning of 2011, the Canadians lead with their factory in Sarina, which produces 97MWp. However, if we were to sum up the locations of the 15 largest solar plants in the world – Europe, led by Germany and followed by Spain and Italy, would be the front-runner. For example, with the solar park in Ammerland, Lower Saxony, Germany became part of the power network generating 21MWp on the 28th of October 2011. Nevertheless, one can but wonder concerning the fact that the park had already been sold on the day of its initiation, in this case to a Hamburg based investment company Aquila Capital. Will human kind really find freedom through renewable energies?

Attached, is a statistic about the 15 largest solar parks in the world (classification 2010):

The 15 largest solar power plants in the world[74]

Output DC (MWp)	Country	Location	Region	Completion
97	Canada	Sarnia	Ontario	2010
84,2	Italy	Montaltodi Castro	Lazio	2010
80,2	Germany	Finsterwalde	Brandenburg	2010
70,6	Italy	San Bellino	Veneto	2010
60	Spain	Olmedillade Alarcón	Kastilien-La Mancha	2008
54	Germany	Straßkirchen	Bavaria	2009
52,8	Germany	Lieberose	Brandenburg	2009
48	USA	BoulderCityNV	Nevada	2010
47,6	Spain	Puertollano	Kastilien-La Mancha	2008
46	Portugal	Amaraleja	Alentejo	2008
42,7	Italy	CellinoSan Marco	Apulien	2010
40	Germany	Brandis	Sachsen	2008
36	Germany	Reckahn	Brandenburg	2010
35	Czech Republic	Vepřek	Středočeský kraj (Mittelböhmen)	2010
34,6	Italy	Sant'Alberto	Emilia-Romagna	2010

Keeping an eye on the near and remote future will be very interesting. The great potential, which lies in the sun energy, is fast being discovered by global markets and will therefore result in rapid developments. It is an exciting topic with a bright future. However, it is necessary to differentiate between countries for which these technologies are reasonable and affordable and those for which they are not.

Humans race after many new developments and like to use nature as their example. Concerning the sun, scientists run tests on nuclear fusion. This simply means the imitation of the sun. Scientists are eager to copy the forces, which make our sun and stars shine within laboratories.

Should these tests be successful and the new source of energy be realized, then many things could change for the human kind. In order for the sun to shine, hydrogen cores have to fuse into helium. This procedure releases unimaginable amounts of energy. However, until those times have arrived, huge obstacles have to be overcome. Atom nuclei can only change into helium at extremely high temperatures above 15 million degrees Celsius.

Up until the reactor catastrophe in 2011 in Fukushima, politics did not show interest in these studies. However, Fukushima moved the global awareness regarding options of energy sources back into the spotlight. The solar power, which we receive from our sun is no other than the harnessed energy produced by nuclear fusion. That energy arrives partly as electromagnetic radiation on Earth. It is a task that raises curiosity because only one second of the energy produced by our sun could cover for all energy demand on Earth until the year 1,002,011. That would of course depend on many different factors on Earth and the human kind over the next million years.

That is also, why a ruling by the German Government to cut the subsidies for a project concerning nuclear fusion was suddenly reversed in April 2011. The Government rediscovered the importance for such projects. Not only Germany showed an immediate interest again in the potential of this research, but also other countries like France and the USA. If the scientists in France are going to be successful with their sophisticated project in Southern France, a version of the fusion could become reality by 2050.

Let us hope all human kind around the world can profit equally from the supply of our sun or the copied laboratory version in future. It is in our hands.

7. Sun Activity and Climate Change

Recently, one of the most delicate themes is of climate change. Are humans to blame because of an excessive output of greenhouse gases, or greedy governments sensing the opportunity for big business from additional emission tax, or are the industries to blame as they use people's fear for their own financial gain, or is it perhaps a very normal natural cycle in solar activity, or will humans enter into a new level of consciousness at about the end of 2012? This is a continued and very interesting debate, which concerns each and every one of us and we should pay some attention.

Some terms will have to be defined before diving into the theme.

Definitions:

Weather (Old High German: wetar = wind, to blow) is a ***short-term*** condition of the atmosphere (also: measurable condition of the troposphere) at a precise location/region on the Earth's surface. It appears in the forms of sunshine, rain, cloud cover, wind, heat or cold.

Meteorology determines the local weather of an exact time on various phenomena in the troposphere, the lower part of the atmosphere. How the weather develops, depends on the atmospheric circulation, which is influenced by the solar radiation and the regional energy balance. Weather means, in a strict sense of the word, a specific condition at a specific location on the Earth's surface, exclusively determined by units of gas pressure, gas density and gas mixture. "Weather" can take place in a laboratory as well as above a continent, without having to alter the definition.[75]

Please note, weather is a ***short-term*** condition, which we can feel, observe and measure during a moment, some minutes, hours or a day in form of wind, rain, heat, cold, clouds etc.

Climate The term climate originates from the Greek word

klimatos = inclination - which means the inclination of the earth´s axis (obliquity of eclipse) against the level of its orbit around the sun.[76] In contrast to the term weather – climate means the condition of the atmosphere and the below lying country or water over *longer* periods. Predictions on climate are usually based on meteorological data. This includes, next to others, the temperature, humidity and atmospheric pressure, wind regime as well as the water temperature above a specific region over a *longer* period. The World Meteorological Organization (WMO) suggests that data of at least 30 years should be evaluated before it is possible to talk about climate.[77]

*Please note: climate are **long-term** observations and measurements of the atmosphere and the country or water lying below – and the consequential statistics arising over many years.*

Climate-variability The term climate-variability mean the climate can change due to *natural* facts independent of human activity. Such external factors are the variation of the intensity regarding the insolation, eruption of volcanos or meteor strikes. Internal factors, however, are based on the variations in the composition of the atmosphere, hydro -, cryo – and biosphere.[78]

*Please note: The climate changes due to **natural** factors.*

Climate change The term climate change is used when mankind directly or indirectly influences the climate. At its center are the emissions of the so-called greenhouse gases (CO_2, CH_4, NO_2 and the chlorine -fluorine-carbonates). Furthermore, climate is influenced by the practice of recovering natural resources, deforestation, the growing urbanization and the changes of land use. Climate change becomes noticeable in forms of cooling or warming of the atmosphere close to the ground.[79]

Please note, climate change is directly or indirectly related to recovering natural resources etc. by humans. Greenhouse gases like CO_2 take up the center.

CO_2 is the chemical formula of carbon dioxide. It is a colorless gas, which is released by burning coal and all organic compounds and it is an end product of the breathing process of people and animals; it is present in the air by _**0.03 percent**_, is absorbed by plants and changed into organic products (carbon cycle).[80]

*Please note, CO_2 is absorbed and transformed by plants. It is contained in the air to **0.03 percent.**_

In the following pages, it will become clear to you why these definitions are important and to what extent they are manipulated. The topic "climate change" is widely discussed with the most diverse opinions, strong provocative theses and far too few honest facts. Furthermore, the facts are manipulated into specific directions pending on the group of interest. All I can recommend for everyone to do is to check carefully the contracting body concerning the line of evidence. Always question their goals and motivations; that way, you will get a little closer to the truth.

Before looking at some of the ambitions of governments, industries and institutions it is important to understand some basic mechanisms of our weather, climate and the sun.

Wind, Clouds, Sun – Weather Ayers Rock, NT, Australia[81]

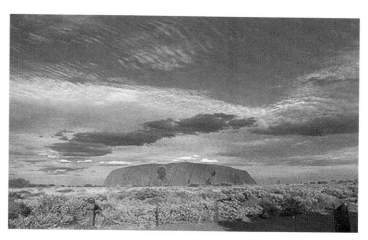

The picture above is representative for our weather, meaning the noticeable, short-term condition of the atmosphere.

Our sun is the engine for our weather. In its deepest core, inner energies are being produced by the process of nuclear fusion, which is released as electromagnetic radiation. The most common form to us is the visible light. Once the solar radiation arrives at the Earth, a hot (close to the equator) or a cold (close to the pole) climate will arise depending on the radiation angle. Our atmosphere arranges the balance of the atmospheric pressure because due to the rising air on the equator (it is warmer) an air deficit on the ground will occur, which we call low-pressure. The opposite happens at the poles, the heavy (cold) air floats down to the ground. To put it more simply, the atmosphere tries to balance the air pressure. Weather is therefore the balancing act of the atmosphere between the contrasts in temperature. In addition to this very simple model, other facts are of importance like vegetation levels, water-land distribution, and rotation of the Earth as well as day – and season rhythms play a part.

Please note: The sun is the engine that drives our weather!

Our intuition gives us a hunch already because, if the sun is indeed the engine for our weather, it might also be the foundation of climate change.

Moreover, indeed never before has the sun been observed by so many objects as today. Scientists are vehemently searching for answers concerning our weather, climate and its changes. To unravel the mystery registering balloons, telescopes, modern satellite technologies, as well as the latest special cameras are being used. It is certain that changes in climate have always existed and cool periods like the ice ages are just as normal as global warming.

The sun has already been verifiably responsible for the diverse climate changes happening on planet Earth during the years 1400 to 1510. The former "Spoerer – Minimum" presented a small ice age, in which the Baltic Sea was completely frozen during winter in 1422/23. At the time, the solar activity was at a minimum and the generation of sunspots widely failed to appear. The same spectacle was repeated during the years 1645 to 1715. This age was also marked by a small ice age called the "Maunder – Minimum". Even the lagoons of Venice formed a thick ice layer during that time. But also the opposite the "warm periods" like the one between 1238 until 1267 are measured. At this time, the temperatures were similarly high compared to today. Therefore, it can be observed that our sun shares the responsibility for our climate change. The sun's strength and effects seem many times larger than has so far been admitted.

A chart published in the Journal of American Physicians and Surgeons concerning the development of the temperature at the surface of the Sargasso Sea shows very clear the cool – and warm periods mentioned before. The temperature varied at about three degrees within the past 3,000 years. It can clearly be seen on the diagram that today's temperatures are even slightly lower than the average in temperature of 23 degrees.

In other words, we are still at the end of a small "ice age" – please see chart:

82

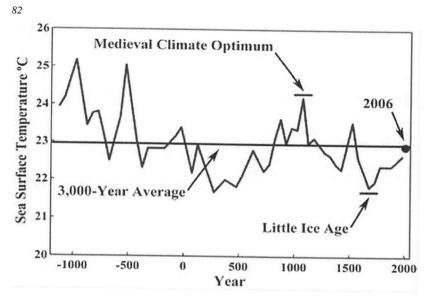

Please note: The sun's responsibility concerning climate changes on Earth is proven for the small ice age 1422/23 and 1645-1715 as well as the warm periods in 1238-1267. Today's temperature is still a little lower compared to the average temperature of the past 3,000 years.

Therefore what exactly is it that is happening on this for us so important star at 150 million kilometers distance?

Scientists have observed the sun did not reach its usual active cycle during the past years. In over 100 years of observation, the sun has never released so little energy as today. The sun, which has been observed constantly since the 18th century, has only had 23 cycles during that time. Due to statistical calculation, the 24th cycle should have started long ago. Usually, such a calm period occurs for no longer than a year due to measurements. However, scientists have been waiting to no avail for the initiation of the activities since 2007. It is also known, that planet Earth had almost no increase in temperature during the past decade. NASA reports the 24th cycle, which we experience at the present, is one of the weakest for 80 years.

The sun is an object, which is constantly moving. The temperatures on the sun's surface are up to 5527 degrees Celsius and in the core up to 15,599,729 degrees Celsius. The temperature on the sunspots is measured at up to 3526 degrees Celsius. Such high temperatures provoke solar eruptions, which can be seen as a bright flash. Scientist's call this process flares with the technical term. Depending on their strength, these flares are able to influence the weather in space and they can reach as far as the Earth. Close to and on our home planet they are able to disrupt sensitive satellites, radios and other transfer mediums. Loss of power would be the worst expected scenario.

The sun is also on the constant move with diverse fields, which rotate at different speeds. This way, in conjunction with magnetic field remains (current occurs), the reversal of the poles is initiated at about every 11 years. Due to calculations by the NASA astronomer David Hathaway, such a solar cycle will take about 131 months with a possible deviation of about 14 months.[83] The average is therefore 11 years. Another very interesting observation by the solar expert David Hathaway shows that the aforementioned current, which is responsible for the cycle of the sunspots, slowed down to a record minimum. This has a huge impact on the future solar activity because scientists assume the speed of the current determines the intensity of the solar spot activity for up to 20 years in advance. A slowed down current means low solar activity. Hathaway believes that the 25th cycle, which peaks in the year 2022 might be one of the weakest in centuries.[84]

The German Heinrich Schwabe discovered the by now well-known eleven - year - solar - cycle as early as the 19th century. Furthermore, it is important to mention the 80 to 90 year lasting Gleissberg – Cycle and the 208-year running de Vries/Suess – Cycle. These cycles can overlap and hence strengthen or weaken the solar activity.

The de Vries/Suess – Cycle is mainly a magnetic activity cycle of the sun. This cycle shows the frequency of occurrence and the extent of the magnetic releases of the sun and the respective connection and influence on our climate and weather. At about 2002/2003 the de Vries/Suess – Cycle had its maximum, when temperatures peaked.[85] The Journal of American Physicians and Surgeons published an illustration concerning the data of the solar activity and the changes in temperature of the past 130 years. This data shows irrepealabl correlations between the solar activity and the changes in temperature.

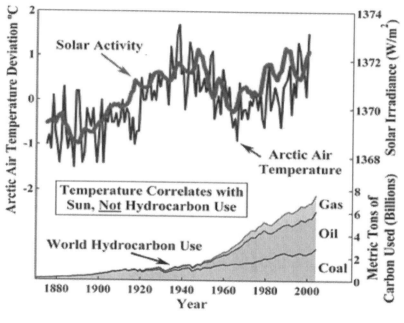

86

Furthermore, there are two very obvious periods. The highest one peaks in the period between 1920 and 1950 at a time when the consumption of coal, gas or oil, and therefore the CO_2 production by humans, was still very remote. There is no evidence between a correlation of the rise in temperature and the CO_2 production. Quite the contrary seems to be the case because at the end of the 60s when the industrialization worked to full capacity the temperatures were rather chilly.

Further very long-term cycles are well known. For example, the orbit of the Earth changes over a period of 100,000 years. The tilt of the Earth´s axis changes every 40,000 years and the phenomenon of whether the northern or southern hemisphere is closer to the sun during summer or winter changes every 25,000 years.

Please note: The sun radiates different levels of energy in diverse cycles (11years, 80-90year and 208years). These cycles can overlap and therefore increase or decrease solar activity. If the activity is higher, it will be warmer on Earth and vice versa. The de Vries/Suess – Cycle had a maximum in about 2002/2003 at which time temperatures peaked.

In easy terms, the extent of our temperature correlates to the solar cycles and their intensity but not to the CO_2 production by humans.

Other scientists believe to have observed the volume of the sun reducing. However, this is very difficult to prove, because the sun moves constantly with bubbles rising up like a boiling pot and the transition into space cannot be exactly distinguished. It is estimated at a range of 300 kilometers. A new French satellite by the name of "Picard" is supposed to bring clarity with the purpose of measuring the diameter of the sun exactly to within a few kilometers. In June 2010, "Picard" was sent into space and we are awaiting exciting results.

During the annual meeting of the European Geophysical Union (EGU) in Vienna in 2009, some participants surprised with little known facts like for example the solar inertial motion (sim) effect. The sun wobbles reportedly permanently around the center of mass of the solar system. Such a "sim – movement" of the sun has an alleged period of 179 year. Hejda Pavel from the Czech Institute for Geophysics in Prague discovered a correlation between such a "sim-period" and volcanic activity.[87]

The fact of the "sim – movement" has been known to astrophysics for decades but it is barely considered in studies or published. Perhaps, we have observed it so far in too few periods and we have forgotten to look at the overall long-term picture. We already know that some centuries ago decreased solar activity led to small ice ages. Back then, those ice ages brought not only cold winters and wet summers but also floods, crop failure and therefore hunger crises.

The sun's part in those ice ages is controversial amongst the scientific community to this day. It is argued that other factors like volcanic activity and sea currents have to be considered as well. However, correlations between volcanic- and solar activity have been discovered by scientists of our times like Hejda Pavel. Natural phenomena like sea currents, the magnetic field and volcanic activity are therefore being influenced by our sun.

The Technical University of Dortmund, Germany published results of a study stating that the solar cycles and cosmic radiation have a much more extensive influence on our climate as has so far been believed. The research is based on measuring data of the past 100 years and has been published in 2010. It seems that the sun changes its average temperature during the course of the before mentioned 11 – year – cycle. If the sun is more active, the temperature will rise and vice versa. During the last 50 years, the sun has had several very active phases and therefore an increased solar - and cosmic radiation.

However, the magnetic fields of the sun turn some of the solar radiation away from the Earth during intense solar - and cosmic radiation. During a solar activity minimum as for instance since 2008, more cosmic radiation will penetrate the atmosphere to reach the Earth. This radiation is first enclosed by air molecules and then by water molecules in the Earth's atmosphere. They either absorb the sunlight or spread it. In other words, less light will reach the Earth´s surface. That is why scientists conclude that the global warming will stagnate in the coming years due to that procedure.[88]

Let us hope the answer to our question of how intense the role of the sun is in regards to our climate change – will find its true meaning in future through objective and independent science. Until then we will blindly trust the technologies of our 21 century, which are very sensitive to solar storms. Should the sun gain full speed in the next months and years (though this is not expected), our space weather will be dramatically influenced. Solar storms, which manage to reach planet Earth, can easily interrupt the sophisticated technologies.

Perhaps, our fantasy can imagine what impact long term power supply failures could do to our supply situation. How quickly will the logistics in the supermarkets come to a standstill? Other scenarios are food supplies, medical supplies, drinking water etc. The American physician has made up his mind: "A solar flare during the years 2012/13 would catapult us back in history for about 100 years."[89] So far, we have been lucky; his prophecy has not come true.

Please note:

A) The 24th solar cycle does not start on time

B) The sun flare activity is less than expected during the past years

C) The magnetic field of the sun weakens

D) The corona changes, meaning changes inside our central celestial body might take place effecting the solar flares

E) Scientist believe in a possible long term decrease in sun spot cycles

F) Correlations between solar activity and volcanic activities, the magnetic field and streaming conditions were discovered

G) Scientists believe that the global warming will stagnate in the years to come

H) The solar activity determines the space weather. Solar storms can reach the Earth and cause interruptions to our sensitive technologies

The listing leads to the quintessence:

__The sun is the motor for the temperatures on Earth, our weather, climate, space weather based on today's knowledge of science and due to long term observations and research.__

We know weather is a short-term occurrence, which can be felt, measured and observed during a moment, minutes, hours or a day in form of wind, rain, heat, chilliness or cloud cover.

We also know the definition of the term climate, which means long-term observations and measurements of the atmosphere and the land or water below and the resulting statistics of this over many years.

We know as well that the sun is the motor for our weather and that changes in temperature on Earth correlate with solar activities, but not with the CO_2 emissions caused by industrialization.

We know furthermore the climate varies due to natural factors.

That is why we should take a very sincere look at the so-called climate change win regards to the human factor. The definition points out that the exploitation of natural resources stands in direct relation to climate change. The greenhouse gases like CO_2 are being discussed in that context as a central point. Let us take a closer look. What are the other factors that exert an influence on our climate and what are the motivations politicians have to fuel this climate hysteria?

A very important resource in this context are our forests. Experts assume one third of the Earth´s surface has been changed by humans. The main reason is seen in forest clearance. The clearance of forest areas has been taken place for about 10,000 years and this can be proven by taking core-drilling samples. China in particular lost huge forest plantations due to rice cultivation. Rice cultivation can be calculated as far back into the past as about 6,000 years. Argentina lost during the past 70 years about 70 percent of their entire forests. In January 2010, the German Ifo Institute reported in a press release on the climate killer deforestation. The global area of forests decreased by three percent between 1990 and 2005.[90] In the past few years, enormous amounts of forest have been cleared in tropical countries (especially Brazil, Indonesia and Sudan). Brazil and Sudan on its own are responsible for 47 percent of the annual global deforestation.[91]

Today, deforestation takes place in Brazil for example, to cultivate soya, sugar cane, palm oil, which is refined into bio-fuel, and used for cattle farming. China, however, has learned from the mistakes made in the past and has contrarily started a large reforestation. China contributes with 73 percent to the annual global growth in forestry.[92]

However, whilst you are reading this book, the deforestation and the total loss of forests will have experienced a rapid rise. This results in the reduction of rainfall and large periods of drought. The Amazon Rainforest was hit by such a drought in the year 2005. The Amazon, which is also called the "green lung", acts as a huge CO_2 (carbon) sink. However, the trees grow more slowly as a result of the droughts and the important effect is regressive. Scientists of the American Duke University in Durham managed to prove the deforestation is in direct correlation to our rainfalls. "Our study had very surprising results, because it showed that the consequences of deforestation had an impact in and close to the related areas but also strong impacts on rainfall in temperate and even higher zones", explains Roi Aviassar, principle author of the research published in the professional journal Hydrometeorology.[93]

The fact is we, and in particular our governments, need to pay a lot more attention to our forests. The World Wide Fund for Nature quotes a study, which calculates that more than half of the Amazon-Forest could be destroyed by 2030, which would result in drastic outcomes regarding the carbon balance.[94] However, the rain forest in the Amazon region is not just essential concerning the CO_2 balance. The research author Dan Nepstad reports that the Amazon is not only essential to cool our planet; it also acts as a large fresh water spring, which could influence ocean currents.[95] Accordingly, our weather will change its well-known patterns due to continued deforestation.

Please note: The forest acts as a CO_2 sink. Rainforests like the Amazon rainforest are essential for the cooling of our planet. They are large fresh water sources, which might even have an impact on ocean currents. However, deforestation steadily continues and half of the Amazon rainforest could be destroyed by 2030. As a result, global weather patterns will change.

Despite those facts, diverse interest groups are fighting amongst each other. On the one hand, there are the so-called climate supporters; it is the group, which claims that the greenhouse gases (CO_2 emissions) produced by humans are responsible for climate change. This can be seen in a report with the title "Review on the Economics of Climate Change" by Professor Sir Nicholas Stern, adviser of the British Government in autumn 2006 concerning economic impacts caused by climate change. Please be reminded of what I wrote before; There is no reliable scientific proof that our CO_2 emissions are responsible for increased temperatures in the atmosphere as currently preached by politicians.

The other group, the climate change skeptics, does not doubt climate change but they see it as a normal phenomenon of nature. That leads us to our next question because what exactly is a normal phenomenon. Is it our weather and climate today or 100 years ago, 1,000 years ago or even 100,000 years ago? That explains why skeptical people are very critical concerning climate change and the subsequent Kyoto – protocol as they can see the controlling attempts of our governments and they believe that controlling our climate by law as absurd.

On 11th December 1997 the Kyoto – protocol was agreed upon; it took the form of an additional protocol to the United Nations framework convention on climate change with the goal to protect the climate. The protocol came into effect on 16th February 2005 and it rules under international law binding aims concerning the emissions of greenhouse gasses in industrialized nations with the justification that this would be the main reason for global warming.[96] [97] The protocol was ratified by 193 states and the European Union up to December 2011.[98] However, Canada announced its disembarkation on the December 13, 2011 and the USA never signed the protocol.[99]

Another climate change skeptic is the Russian Academy of Science, which published a report as early as 2004 stating that the emissions, which are produced by humans, are insignificantly small compared to the total greenhouse effect. Additionally, Fritz Vahrenholt, former senator of environment, Hamburg and today's chairman of RWE-Innology, and Sebastian Luening, geologist, point out in their book "Die kalte Sonne, The cold sun" that the portion of carbon dioxide on our climate could be disregarded.

Ever-increasing amounts of scientists believe the CO_2 is to blame for our climate warming. The portion of carbon dioxide (CO_2) in our atmosphere is only 0.03 percent. These already show how nonsensical the thesis concerning CO_2 possibly being the only explanation for global warming really is.[100] At the annual meeting of the European Geophysical Union (EGU) in Vienna in April 2009 which 8,000 geo-scientists attended, the following question was raised and intensely debated: "If and how planet movements and solar activity impact on climate change as well as other geological proceedings on Earth."[101] This then is where the loop closes because by looking back at the consolidated findings this question can already be answered by using available science and observations.

Please note: Scientists disbelieve that the greenhouse gases (CO_2 emissions) are the only reason on which to blame the change in climate. They argue that the CO_2 portion with as little as 0.03 percent in the atmosphere is too small to have an impact.

However, the World Climate Council IPCC sees it in a different way.

The 4th report of the World Climate Council IPCC, which was published in 2007, draws a very controversial scenario. This report states that humans and their production of CO_2 emissions are responsible for the prognosticated climate change. The report warns about rising temperatures on Earth and subsequently droughts in Africa and Southern Europe, floods in the river deltas and the loss of fertile land in Asia, heavy rainfalls and storms in North Europe, the shrinking of the Greenland – and polar ice, etc. The list of horror scenarios, for which humans are responsible, is long.

The reports of the IPCC are meant to be the scientific base for international climate politics. The interstate expert advisory board for climate change (IPCC) was founded by the international community of states in 1988 in order to analyze the latest results on global climate science. The IPCC is a scientific body, which does not accomplish any scientific research work itself.[102] Many of its published fundamentals and recommendations are based on results, which are entirely based on model calculations. And that is, where the problem occurs. We cannot understand the total complexity of all proceedings in nature and their details at full length. For that reason, simplified models are created by scientists in comparison to reality, to establish and forecast principles and behavior patterns. In order to be able to use these models in a practical way, they have to be scientifically approved before use in terms of completeness, accuracy and their scope of application. In this regard, scientific proof for the base of our climate models is missing even today and therefore the calculated results are very questionable. Such model calculations can hardly refute scientific data and facts, which are gained from reality.

In the past, as a matter of fact, reports by the IPCC have shown mistakes and inaccuracies. However, these reports are the base foundation for political decisions. For example, the 4th progress report was reviewed by experts regarding its accuracy. Mistakes and inaccuracies could be proven, which resulted in strong criticism for the IPCC. In order to prevent mistakes in the reports a reform process was initiated and a review committee founded by the United Nations (UN) and the World Climate Council in 2010. This way the quality of the reports is meant to improve and the trust of the public shall be rehabilitated.[103]

Let's have a look at a current example from May 2012. The University of Melbourne conducted a research project concerning climate warming. The research, led by Dr. Joelle Gergis and co-authors, was published in May 2012 and engaged in the rise in temperature in Australia and bordering regions.[104]

An American by the name of Michael Mann distinguished the "hockey stick theory" in the late 1990s and the scientists in Australia stated the same theory applied to Australia. It says that the temperatures have risen only significantly since the industrial age.

The new research results spread like wildfire in Magazines, on TV and in scientific articles. Even the 5th report of the IPCC aimed to include this data in order to underline its model calculations. But far wrong – the research, which was planned from mid-2009 to mid-2012 at as reported by media a total value of 950,000 dollar, could keep the pot boiling for just about three weeks. In a detailed analysis, the study discovered that Australia and its neighboring regions had only experienced a rise in temperature of 0.09 degrees Celsius (meaning it is absolutely within normal range) compare to the reference period of 1,000 years. This is based on observations of tree groups in Tasmania and in New Zealand. Steve McIntyre, a diligent statistician, had a go on the study and uncovered serious methodic – and mathematical mistakes within the statistical analysis. Meanwhile, the paper vanished from many web pages like the Journal of Climate.[105]

The question of how such mistakes are still possible after the implementation of a review committee by the IPCC has to be raised. This can only be answered by keeping the numerous interest groups, who do not want to lose their benefits gained from the new climate religion, in mind.

Let us have a quick recap of the 4th IPCC – Report (AR4) by task group III. Diverse models concerning the reduction of global warming to 2.0 to 2.4°C compared to the pre-industrial age are being discussed (2° goal). Center of the discussion is the long-term stabilization of atmospheric greenhouse gas emissions. Measures from all economic sectors are determined – energy, transport, buildings, industry, agriculture and forestry as well as waste management.

However, beware, because the UK Met Office revised its previous models and announced in December 2012 that older models are wrong. Against all odds, the results show that the global temperature has stagnated (observed from 1997 to the present) and that this could continue to at least 2017, meaning a 20-year period of no statistically significant change in global temperature.

This shows once more, how easy the model calculations of the IPCC can begin to falter. To date, the master plan of our climate remains a mystery to science. However, our media and governments accept unquestioningly the model based predictions. Perhaps, the so-called skeptics are actually on the right track after all!

However, the bourgeois of Australia have made up their minds in September 2013. The last Government Elections in September has been seen on a par with a referendum concerning carbon tax and Emission trading. The vast majority of the population voted against those taxes and for a new Government under the Liberal Party chaired by Tony Abbott. The newly elected Premier gave notice to the „Australian Climate Commission", this being one of his first acts. He was quoted in the media with the words that climate change was a complete load of garbage. [106] It is also emphasized that countries, in which carbon tax is payable, are at risk of economical shortfalls.

Please note: The reports of the global climate council (IPCC) state humans and their produced emissions are to blame for the climate change. It is proven that the reports of the IPCC contain mistakes.

At the beginning of this chapter, I made you aware that it is important to keep an eye on some interest groups and to challenge their argumentation in order to edge a little closer to the truth.

We should take a look at politics in this respect. During the past years, many states introduced carbon taxes and politics would favor a global tax in the case of CO_2. So, this tax has allegedly become inevitable in Australia in 2012. The country was faced with severe natural catastrophes in 2011, which resulted in crop failures and a decrease in the tourist industry. Despite strong doubts regarding the theory of manmade warming by David Evans, climate scientist of the Australian Department of Climate Warmth, there was no compromise concerning the tax. The mining industry booms in these parts of the Earth like never before and the demand for raw materials as gold, natural gas, rare ores, uranium and coal is large and as is the aligned environmental damage. The largest coral reef on Earth the Great Barrier Reef at the coastline of Australia has been adversely affected by the mining industries. In 1981, it was declared a world natural heritage and it one of the seven wonders of nature. The reef is located at the East Coast of Queensland and extends along a length of about 2,400 km. It is located in the South Pacific and runs almost parallel along the East Coast at a distance of about 30 to 250 km (between Cairns and Gladstone) and measures an area of 347,800 km². [107] The reef has an invaluable wealth of marine animals, plants and sea birds. Despite the coral reef being a highly sensitive ecological system, the construction work at the harbor in Gladstone continues undeterred. The mining industry uses the harbor to export raw materials, especially the precious natural gas. The shipping industry has significantly increased in the region of the reef and will continue to grow in the coming years.

This example should show that we care little about our environment but our global world seems spot on when it comes to taxes concerning the alleged climate change. It seems as if there are two different rules concerning climate warming and the general environmental protection.

___The fact is___ if we carry on destroying our environment systematically and with sophisticated technologies at ever increasing speed by the uncontrolled exploitation of raw materials and natural resources to produce perishables and cheap non-durable goods, which we return to nature in the form of rubbish, which then destroys the rest of our environment, a discussion around the alleged climate change is absurd. The wealth, which will be lost in the case of the reef, is inconceivable for humanity.

Let's look at two more examples concerning the handling of the clime change from a German perspective. Germany drew a strange picture concerning the climate at the UN-climate summit in Copenhagen end of 2009.

The two chief editors of the two most influential German Media outlets ARD and ZDF (Channel one and two German TV News) protested in a letter, dating 17.12.2009, against the massive restrictions of independent news coverage at the UN-climate summit in Copenhagen. The letter was addressed to the German chancellor Angela Merkel, the Federal Minister of Foreign and Environmental Affairs, the Danish Premier Lars Rasmussen and the UNO-Agencies in Bonn and New York. The letter reads: "Journalists are not allowed to move freely within the conference center. Spontaneous shoots are impossible."[108]

All too often climate change was designated for political use. Before now, the former German chancellor Schmidt defended the development of nuclear power engineering with the argument: "I do not want our grandchildren to choke on carbon dioxide. It is obvious to any ordinary person that nuclear power stations do not produce carbon dioxide unlike coal-burning power plants."[109]

Isn´t it interesting that the former chancellor justified the introduction of nuclear power plants with the argument of climate change and the officiating chancellor renewed the contract periods for nuclear power plants in 2010. Only a few months later the same chancellor put Germany's energy politics on hold – what happened to change her mind so rapidly? The answer is the sad events following the tsunami in Japan, where a power station was damaged so badly by the high impact radioactivity was released. Thousands of people will never be able to return to their homes as a result.

Another example comes from the USA. The American president was rewarded a Nobel Peace Prize out of the blue in 2009. The media's reaction was surprise and they asked - for what? – For peace or climate protection? Maybe, the prize came too early after merely a year in office. Barack Obama, who was busy at the time discussing the war operation in Afghanistan, was complimented by the committee for a "new climate in world politics".[110]

He was also praised for his serious commitment to climate change prevention. An article published on the 9. October 2009 just before the climate summit reads as follows: "The US government will arrive at the climate summit in Copenhagen in December with a deadlocked draft bill concerning the limitation of pollutant emissions and the facilitation of renewable energies."[111] No wonder then, the media asked what the Nobel Peace Prize was for. The answer might be that the president had a very low survey rating at the time and something had to happen to promote him.

Please note:

Change in climate – justifies the implementation of additional tax sources

Change in climate – justifies transformations in energy politics

Change in climate – used for political image improvement

Media coverage was restricted at the climate summit in

Copenhagen

By looking at the examples listed above, the strong suspicion emerges that not everything is handled reputably concerning climate change.

As demonstrated in the previous pages, it can be concluded that our sun and diversely changed circumstances on Earth like the use of land (deforestation) are responsible for our weather, climate and climate change.

That is where the question arises, if the manmade portion of CO_2 pollution is not responsible for the long-term climate change why are we being frightened and horrified with reports like the 4th IPCC?

Nigel Calder, former editor of the New Scientist abstracts the subject with the following words: "The business with the Earths warming has become a type of religion. Who disagrees is a heretic."

The propaganda of the new religion called global warming is so intense people are afraid to voice a different opinion. It is seen as good, commendable and correct to campaign for climate protection. Unfortunately, the term climate protection is falsely interpreted and associated in peoples mind with the term global warming due to manmade CO_2 emissions. And that is why people are being charged exaggerated cots of energy, climate protecting products or tax. They are asked or forced to use too expensive light bulbs or to insulate their homes repeatedly. In Germany an energy passport for houses was introduced, the rubbish has to be thoroughly sorted the heating facilities have to be changed into climate friendly ones and, of course, not to forget, there is the CO_2 emissions in cars.

A much more efficient solution would be to reduce the CO_2 portion in the atmosphere by implementing the immediate stop of uncontrolled deforestation and the reforestation of such regions. This way, much more could be achieved in the long run than by all the other listed scenarios.

The industries' business booms as never before due to climate fears.

The business with climate fear allows industries to boom as never before and so does the CO_2 emission trading. APA Copenhagen announced in a report from March 2008: "The trade with CO_2 emissions in order to reduce greenhouse gases is globally raised by 80 percent to a value of 40 billion Euros..."[112] Here too, it is a very prospering business.

We in the industrialized states are not the only ones that are made to pay, but people are also being soaked in the Third World, where the CO_2 lie is just as present. Africa, which is rich in natural resources like coal and crude oil, is forced into alternative energy's like solar - and wind power by climate protection measures. These are energies, which many of the developing countries are unable to effort. No matter which motives are perused, the losers are always the ones that have to pay - no matter whether it is in the First - or Third World.

Please note: We are all being made to pay by playing up the anxiety of rising temperatures, which are verifiably within limits, and the myth of the manmade climate change. The CO_2 lie is as obvious as never before.

The suns activities cannot be controlled by human laws and our future lies, sort of, in the stars. However, mass deforestation, mass contamination of our oceans and many of the secret projects could be controlled by legislation and consequent measures.

The power obsessed human plays with fire and would like to control natural laws. The HAARP-project in Alaska is an example to support the experimentation claim. An online article describes the project with the following content: "The so-called HAARP-project (High Frequency Active Auroral Research Program) heats up the ionosphere with gigantic energy guzzlers (up to 100 billion watt) in order to affect the Earth's surface and human consciousness with the help of the notorious ELF-waves. They can globally and exactly ... transfer cancer information or other disease related information. It is possible to drive a complete town insane, the weather can be influenced, the terrestrial pole can be moved, earthquakes can be triggered etc. There is almost nothing that could not be done by that technology."[113]

This is an example of current speculations. This research can be found on a global scale. They are mainly financed by the militaries and therefore us taxpayers. Many conspiracy theories and speculations exist. However, the plain real truth could be one, which is mind-blowing.

For a long time, humans have played with the idea of controlling our weather. It is assumed that 20 percent of all airplane condensation trails are not such, but are, in fact, so called "chemtrails". The name derives from the appearance and substances of these unbelievable and uncontrolled spray- and emission activities from planes.[114]

Reportedly, chemicals are emitted into the atmosphere from military – and civil planes with the idea of diminishing the solar radiation and therefore global warming. It is said the chemicals, which are sprayed, are harmful aluminum and barium oxides in the form of Nano particles. The purpose of those sprayings has not been fully established because there is no explicit feedback from governmental departments. Weather manipulation or military exercises are suspected to be behind the sprayings. We humans can distinguish the trails from normal plane trails by the characteristic of their durability. Real trails will disappear from the skies after a few minutes or, depending on the air temperature and humidity, might last up to 30 minutes. Chemtrails remain during the course of the day and finally change into a milky appearance.[115]

It is assumed these tests are subject to the utmost secrecy as the negative effects of such uncontrollable sprayings have not yet been researched and calculated fully. The consignors do not want to be liable for the risks that may occur from such experiments. Despite long term environmental damages, increased fire danger in forests through sediments and other problems like Alzheimer, respiratory disease and allergies in humans may occur due to the spreading of these chemicals. Despite the denials of such tests by our governments, it is astonishing that a new patent in conjunction with aluminum tolerant plant gene was registered (see United States Patent 7,582,809 1.September, 2009).

To seek justifications for such practices, the finger is all too often pointed to the alleged manmade climate change. For a long time now, has it been used as a magic-cap for spooky experiments to control the weather and therefore mankind? People agree frivolously when they are made to believe it for the saving of the climate.

The chemtrails are only a small section of possible scenarios, which are under way to control our weather. The more official version states it is all about reducing CO_2.

The CO_2 fabrication and the alleged need for reducing the global CO_2 are only cover-ups. During the last few years, many patents concerning highly technical interventions in the climate system are being registered. Terms like geo-engineering and climate engineering are being used. The Federal Government of Germany defines the buzzword as follows: "Geo-engineering (or Climate-Engineering) is targeted, large scaled technical interventions of humans into the climate/the climate events. It is split into two procedural methods: the management of solar irradiation in order to cool the Earth artificially and the removal of carbon from the atmosphere. ..."[116]

Some artificial methods to reduce carbon from the atmosphere and to influence the solar irradiation are being discussed:

- Reflectors in space
- Ocean fertilization (already tested and done by Germany)
- Insertion of aerosols into the stratosphere (for example as fuel additive in passenger planes)
- Clouds will be artificially changed or dissolved
- The surface of the Earth shall get a new shiny look (as e.g. with white roofs or shiny plants)
- Carbon deposition in oceans, acceleration of ocean ventilation (CO_2 will be discharged into deeper layers)
- Manipulation of natural decomposition processes
- Biological techniques for marine carbon absorption (algae growth)
- Chemical carbon filtration from air
- Biological techniques for absorbing and depositing carbon (reforestation of savannahs)

What sounds like science fiction is, unfortunately, the bitter reality. Experts do not doubt the implementation of these designs can cause unpredictable damages to our environments, which change all our lives forever. A tide of patents was registered concerning the aforementioned methods during the past years. Large cooperation's like Shell, Microsoft (Bill Gates) assist in financing diverse projects. It is served up to us as part of the menu of climate change but it might be indigestible for all living creatures. The aforementioned technologies are only being discussed in connection with the alleged climate warming and nobody seems to be aware of the obvious possibilities regarding these destructive technologies for military operations like weapons of mass destruction (WMD). However, it gets worse because our entire food chain would be struck by such technologies as well as the balance of all on Earth occurring natural processes.

The media and intelligence services like to blame terrorism and rogue regimes as threats to civilization, but the truth is that the biggest threat is posed by the aggressive and reckless destruction of our natural resources, and therefore our natural balance. Dr. Rosalie Bertell writes in her book "Planet Earth. The Latest Weapon of War" that annually 422 million hectares of ecological resources are wasted for the production of weapons in the United States, Russia, China, Great Britain, France, Germany and Japan.[117]

How meaningless would a war for humanity be, if there was no clean air or clear drinking water, and if the fields could no longer be tilled? The all above listed technologies have the power to trigger an avalanche of such a scenario. Human kind has no more time to waste.

The Australian weekly newspaper `Die neue Woche´ published an article on March 4th, 2014 concerning some research on the manipulation of the global climate. German scientists from Kiel, David Keller and Prof. Oschlies state that climate – engineering methods are little efficient and dangerous. Once such methods are introduced, they cannot be stopped, without speeding up change climate.[118] "Prof Oschlies told the German Press Association that the focus on climate – engineering science is the USA, Great Britain and Canada: „Their feasibility studies are taking place, the technical implementation …"In order to shade sunlight it is possible that Aerosol-Trails will be launched in the USA this year. "That is very widely, very really planned."[119]

The tip of the iceberg is, in their professional article, German Scientists from Kiel mention that even the combination of various climate – engineering technologies could NOT reduce global warming. To reach the goal of limiting the rise in temperature by 2 degrees Celsius by 2100 is said to be impossible. The technologies of climate – engineering are said to be relatively ineffective in relation to warmth reduction (less than 8 percent), and the experts warn about dangerous side effects.

We should ask ourselves seriously, if such methods have no or only an insignificant impact on climate warming, why are they being discussed and implemented? These trails are very dangerous. Why are they being conducted despite warnings from scientists? What is their real target and purpose?

One day, hopefully not too late for the human kind, the truth be revealed? Until then, we might witness many more alleged natural phenomena, like the mass stranding of whales in New Zealand in early 2011, in Japan in April 2012 and currently in Port Macquarie, Australia. Suddenly, flocks of migratory birds fall out of the skies, increased tsunamis and earthquakes, droughts as well as floods. January 2014 also saw destructive floods in England on an unprecedented scale, 10-meter high monster waves on Portugal's coastline, sudden falls in temperature by 30 degrees and a snow chaos in North America, spring like warm temperatures during the winter months in Germany and extensive droughts in Australia. Simultaneously with the monster waves in Portugal, thousands of flying foxes fell from the skies in the Hinterland of the Sunshine Coast in Queensland. The local council blamed the heat as a cause for the dead bats.

International climate politics has defined a so-called "two degree goal". It means that the global warming has to be limited to less than two degrees compared to the levels from before the beginning of industrialization. It is important for us to understand that our current temperatures, despite the global warming of the past decades, *are still below* the maximum temperatures of the past 2000 years from before industrialization. The in the mainstream media widely discussed "two degree goal" is to this effect not even bothered. We are still within the natural belt of fluctuation. Therefore, the question of who profits from all the reasons of precaution and the already implemented gigantic multi-billion Dollar schemes arises.

Maybe, the natural climate cycles will indeed soon be imbalanced, caused by dangerous climate engineering trials, like feared by the previously quoted scientists from Kiel in Germany.

Humans chase after projects, which can easily get out of control and they are therefore irresponsible. Meanwhile, the ordinary innocent citizen will be blamed for changed climate conditions and will be asked to pay.

Fundamental and existential things like our natural basis to our sun and therefore our light and our well-being are not being presented in the right light. This is essential information for us to enable us to make the correct decisions. These decisions are fundamental for securing our- and the future for generations to come. They are important for a healthy and happy life.

Our sun is an essential factor. It keeps endless processes running on our home planet Earth. We should all have the basic right to be enlightened in an honest manner and to a full extent. It would be right to take a closer look at our sun in order to lift its mysteries and consequences. To do so, political, military and industrial as well as wrongly motivated and ambitioned driving power should stay in the background [120]for the collective good and the survival of human kind.

Our native ancestors knew about the great influence and power of the sun. They lived with the sun and the nature in balanced harmony. For example, the Aboriginal people of Australia saw themselves as a part of nature and they have kept that wisdom for more than 60,000 years. They lived in balance with their environment and the elements. They saw themselves as a part herein and not as the over man. Modern time's superman aims to enslave the nature, climate, weather and therefore our human race!

"A WISE HUMAN RESPECTFULLY PERCEIVES

HIS ENVIRNOMENT, FELLOW MEN,

SUN-SYSTEM, UNIVERSE,

AND HIMSELF AS A WHOLE"

Elisabeth J. Ellmer

About the Author

The author preferably publishes controversial non-fiction literature. Her involvement with the main stream media for over two decades leads to her unusual life experience, which provides the foundation for her research. The open minded author remains curious and cautious about current affairs. She publishes "books with perspectives". The native German lives in her adopted country Australia.

www.jutta-ellmer.com
www.sunenergetics.com

Elisabeth J. Ellmer

Preliminary Note of Use:

This book was researched with extraordinary diligence, and references are used in good conscience.

However, the evidence provided does not replace any professional, medical, psychological or technical advice.

Each reader is responsible for their own handling of the do's and the don'ts. Neither the author nor the publisher or people involved in the production of this book or those named intend to diagnose or recommend any kind of therapy.

No liabilities will be considered concerning possible disadvantages or damages resulting from practical or theoretical references within the book.

You are responsible!

Elisabeth J. Ellmer

Dictionary

Basal-cell carcinoma (BCC), white skin cancer

Chlorophyll, leaf green

Chronobiology, anatomy of the rhythms

Daylight saving, clock change winter/summer

HAARP, High Frequency Active Auroral Research Program

Heliotherapy, Light therapy

Jetlag, tiredness after long distance flights

Colonoscopy, bowel screening

Malign melanoma, dark/black skin cancer

Sol, Soll, Sunna, Sonne, sun

Solar, concerning the sun

Sun globule, sugar balls, which are enriched with the sun's spectrum

Stromatolithe, algae mat (Australia)

Sunna, sun goddess

Suray Namaskar, sun salutation yoga

Elisabeth J. Ellmer

Abbreviations

BAD, British Association of Dermatologists

BAG, Federal Office of Health (Switzerland)

CFC, chlorofluorocarbon

IACR, International Agency of Cancer Research

IU, IE, International Units/Einheiten

IPCC, Intergovernmental Panel on Climate Change

PV, photovoltaic

RA, color rendering

Ri, color index

SDO, Solar Dynamic Observatory

UBA, Federal Environmental Agency

UV, ultraviolet

WHO, World Health Organization

ZVEI, German Federation of Electrical Engineering and Industry

Elisabeth J. Ellmer

References

[1] http://de.wikipedia.org/wiki/Stonehnege translation J.E.

[2] www.lokis-mythologie.de/Sunna.html

[3] Bundesanstalt für Arbeitsschutz und Arbeitsmedizin. Geringer Eigenschutz der Haut vor UV Strahlung. 12.08.2010

[4] Bayerisches Landesamt für Umwelt, Referat 12 – Infozentrum Umwelt Wissen, Verfasserin Ulrike Koller März 1993, Überarbeitung Dr. Katharina Stroh Juni 2002, Links 2005

[5] http://www.bom.gov.au/uv/2011

[6] C. Garbe (Hrsg.): Interdisziplinäre Leitlinien zur Diagnostik und Behandlung von Hauttumoren, Thieme Verlag 2005
R.M. Szeimies, A. Hauschild, C. Garbe, R. Kaufmann, M. Landtaler (Hrsg.): Tumoren der Haut: Grundlagen – Diagnostik – Therapie, Thieme Verlag 2010
H.-J. Schmoll, K. Höffken, K. Possinger (Hrsg.): Kompendium Internistische Onkologie, Springer Verlag 2006
Robert Koch-Institut (Hrsg.) Krebs in Deutschland 2005/2006. Häufigkeiten und Trends, Berlin 2010

[7] Gesetz zur Regelung des Schutzes vor nichtionisierender Strahlung (/gesetze_verordnungen/bmu-downloads/doc/print/44925.php) 03.08.2009

[8] E.T. Wolf and O.B. Toon. Fractal Organic Hazes provided an Ultraviolet Shield for Early Earth. Science, 4 June 2010: Vol. 328. no. 5983, pp. 1266 – 1268 DOI: 10.1126/science.1183260

[9] Dr. Rosalie Bertell. Kriegswaffe Planet Erde. Page 148 Issue 12/2011

[10] „Environment News Service Daily", 13 February 1992. Kriegswaffe Planet Erde. Dr. Rosalie Bertell. P. 148 Issue 12/2011

[11] K.M. Hanson et al., Sunscreen enhancement of UV-induces reactive oxygen species in the skin, Free Radic Biol Med.;41(8):1205-12

[12] Health Research Forum Occasional Reports: No 1. Sunlight Robbery. Oliver Gillie

[13] Jacob Liberman, Natürliche Gesundheit für die Augen Sehstörungen beheben, die Sehkraft verbessern, Integral 1997

[14] European Journal of Clinical Nutrition (2008) 62, 1079-1089; doi:10.1038/sj.ejcn.1602825; published online 30 May 2007

[15] Hintzpeter B, et al. Zitat 3: Eigenschaft des Vitamin D im Kindesalter. Proceedings of the German Nutrition Society 10 2007; 10:47.

[16] ScienceDaily, May 19, 2011. Sun Protects Against Childhood Asthma

[17] Nature Reviews Edocrinology 7, 337-345 (June 2011) / doi:10.1038/nrendo.2010.226

[18] ABC News Australia.26.07.2011 Interview with Prof.Peter Ebeling. Western Health Service. Low vitamin D levels linked to diabetes risk.

[19] Brenner H, et al.; Eight years of colonoscopic bowel cancer screening in Germany: initial findings and projections. Dtsch Arztebl Int 2010; 107(43): 753-9

[20] Eickhoff A, Hartmann D, Striegel J and Riemann JF, „Früherkennung und Primärpräventation des Dickdarmkrebses", Der Onkologe 2008;14(2):131-141

[21] Atlas of cancer mortality in the United States, 1950-94. Washington DC:US Govt Print Off 1999 (NIH publ.No (NIH) 99-4564)).

[22] Studie: Johan Moan et al., Colon Cancer: Prognosis for different latitudes, age groups and seasons in Norway, Journal of Photochemistry and Photobiology, 89, 2007, 148-155

[23] Studie: Song-Yi Park et al., Calcium and Vitamin D Intake and Risk of Colorectal Cancer: The Multiethnic Cohort Study, American Journal of Epidemiology, 2007, 165:784-793

[24] Studie: Silvia Alvarenz-Diaz et al., Cystatin D is a candidate tumor supressor gene induced by vitamin D in human colon cancer cells, Journal of Clinical Investigation, July 2009

[25] BMG, BMU, Kooperationsgemeinschaft Mammographie

[26] ENCR Cancer Fact Sheets, Vol.2, Dec.2002

[27] www.who.int/mediacentre/factsheets/fs297/en/

[28] Studienbericht – MARIE-Studie Version 1.3_23.03.2009

[29] http://photomed.wordpress.com/2007/02/02/441/

[30] www.reuters.com/article/idUSTRE63S4GH20100429

[31] West Australian, 18/10, p13; Adelaide Advertiser, p6

[32] Parkin DM, Bray F, Ferlay J. Pisani P. Global cancer statistics, 2002. CA Cancer J Clin 2005;55(2):74-108

[33] Grumet SC, Bruner DW, The identification and screening of men at high risk for developing prostate cancer. Urol Nurs 2000;20:15-8,23-4,46.

[34] http://www.gesundheitsseiten.com/indikationen-l-z/27-indikationen-l-z/157-prostatakrebs.html

[35] EUROPEANJOURNALOFCANCER42(2006) 2222-223H.J. von der Rheea,

*, E. de Vriesb, J.W.W. Coeberghb,c

aDepartment of Dermatology, Leyenburg Hospital, P.O. Box 40551, Leyweg 275, 2504 LN Den Haag, Zuid-Holland, The Netherlands

bDepartment of Public Health, Erasmus MC, P.O. Box 1738, 3000 DR Rotterdam, The Netherlands

cEindhoven Cancer Registry, Comprehensive Cancer Centre South, P.O. Box 231, 5600 AE Eindhoven, The Netherlands

[36] Bodiwala D, Luscombe CJ, French ME, et al. Associations between prostate cancer susceptibility and parameters of exposure to ultraviolet radiation. Cancer Lett 2003;200:141-8.

[37] John EM, Schwartz GG, Koo J. Van Den Berg D, Ingles SA. Sun exposure, vitamin D receptor gene polymorphisms, and risk of advanced prostate cancer. Cancer Res 2005;65:5470-9.

[38] www.weltbevoelkerung.de. 13.03.2013

[39] www.destatis.de. 04.09.2011

[40] www.drstrunz.de/news/2009/12/100104_vitamind.php

[41] Published online 2 July 2007 in Wiley InterScience (www.interscience.wiley.com) DOI:10.1002/dmrr.737. Correlation between vitamin D3 deficiency and insulin resistance in pregnancy. Zhila Maghooli. Arash Hossein-nezhad. Farzaneh Karimi. Ali-Reza Shafaei. Bagher Larjani

[42] European Journal of Clinical Nutrition (2009) 63, 473-477. Association of subclincal vitamin D deficiency in newborns with acute lower respiratory infection and their mothers. G Karatekin, A Kaya. Ö Salihogulu. H Balci. A Nuhoglu

[43] http://www.medivere.de/blog/wp-content/uploads/40813_zusammenfassung_lunch_symposium_vitamind.pfd

[44] Quelle: Oh J et al. 1,25(OH)2 vitamin D inhibits foam cell formation and suppresses macrophage cholesterol uptake in patients with type 2 diabetes mellitus. Circulation 120: 687-698, 2009; doi: 10.1161/circulationsaha. 109.856070

[45] Eva Ellmer, B.Ex&SpSci(Hons), AEP, ESSAM, 2014

[46] http://naturheilkundelexikon.de/glossar/chronobiologie.php

[47] http://www.landlive.de/blogs/entries/623/

[48] Reiter u. Robinson, „Melatonin", page 241

[49]http://de.wikipedia.org/w/index.php?title=Datei:Photosynthese_Lichtmenge.sv g&filetimestamp=20091013130551.Urheber.Yikrazuul

[50] http://superchlorophyll.blogspot.com/

[51]„Gesundheitswunder Chlorophyll – Gespeicherte, gesundheitsspendende Sonnen- und Heilkraft" G.A. Ulmer S. 54-58

[52] Bohn T, Walczyk S, Leisibach S, Hurrell RF. Chlorophyll-bound magnesium in commonly consumed vegetables and fruits: relevance to magnesium nutrition. J Food Sci. 2004;69(9):S347-S350

[53] Min Chen, Martin Schliep, Robert Willows, Zheng-Li Cai, Brett A. Neilan, Hugo Scheer; „A red-shifted chlorophyll"; Science online, 19. August 2010

[54] Linda Jenkins, Australia, Montville, 2013

[55] Ott, John Nash, School Lighting and Hyperactivity, Journal for Biosocial Research, Summer 1980, page 6-7 / Ott, John Nash Influence of Fluorescent Light and Learning Disabilities, Journal of Learning Disabilities, August – September 1976, page 417-422

[56] Hollwich, Fritz and Dieckhues, B., The Effect of Natural and Artificial Light via the Eye on the Hormonal and Metabolic Balance of Animal and Man, Ophthalmologica, 1980, Vol. 180, no 4, page 188-197

[57] http://www.netzmafia.de/skripten/hardware/Licht/index.html. 04.09.2012

[58] www.oekotest.de ÖKO-Test Online Testberichte Energiesparlampen

[59] www.dailymail.co.uk/health/article-506082/Environmentally-friendly-light-bulbs-skin-cancer.html

[60] http://www.energystar.gov/index.cfm?fuseaction=find_a_product.showProductGroup&pgw_code=LB.13.06.2011

[61] U.S. Government Printing Office: Public Law 110 – 140 – Energy Independence and Security Act of 2007 (http:/www.gpo.gov/fdsys/pkg/PLAW-110publ140/content-detail.html)

[62] WORLD RESOURCE REWVIEW, VOL 12, 12, NOS 2-4 – GLOBAL WARMING SCIENCE & POLICY, PTS 1-3 : 717-731 2000

[64] „Die Woche" Volume No. 5.page 10. Staaten einig über Konvention zur Quecksilber-Reduzierung. 29.01.2013

[65] Stellungnahme des Umweltbundesamtes zu angeblichen Phenol-und Aromatendämpfen aus Energiesparlampen vom 21. April 2011

[66] www.bag.admin.ch/aktuell/00718/01220/index.html?lang=de&msg-id=32450

[67] www.buergerwelle-scheiz.org/lampen.505.0.html

[68] www.oekotest.de ÖKO-TEST Online Testberichte Energiesparlampen

[69] www.elektrofachkraft.de/fachwissen/fachnews/kritik-an-energiesparlampen

[70] http://www.photovoltaic-production.com/4552/robust-pv-installation-growth-prodicted-for-2013/

[71] GTM Research (Cambridge, Massachusetts, USA) 2011.

[72] http://solarserver.de/solar-magazin/nachrichten/aktuelles/2011/kw07/gtm-research-weltmarkt-der-photovoltaik-materialien-waechst-bis-2014-um-50.html

[73] Bundesministerium für Wirtschaft und Technologie Stand: 25. Oktober 2012

[74] http://www.solarserver.de/service-tools/statistics-und-markforschung/photovoltaik/maerkte.html

[75] http://14-tage-wettervorhersage.de/allgemein/wetter-wikipedia/

[76]
http://www.dwd.debvbw/appmanager/bvbw/dwdwwwDesktop?_nfpb=true&_pageLabel=_dwdwww_spezielle_nutzer_schule_klima&T25800141921160367837390gsbDocumentPath=Navigation%2FOeffentlichkeit%2FSpezelle_Nutzer%2FSChulen%2FKlima%2FBegriffe%2FKlima_node.html%3F_nnn%3Dtrue

[77] http://www.excha.de/laintro.htm Abs. 1

[78] http://www.excha.de/laintro.htm Abs.2

[79] http://www.excha.de/laintro.htm Abs.3

[80] Meyers großes Handlexikon.15.Auflage.Seite 452

[81] Armin Ellmer, Pilot, 2012

[82] Robinson A.B., Robinson N.E., and Soon W.: Environmental effects of increased atmospheric Carbon Dioxide. Journal of American Physicians and Surgeons, 12/2007, 79-90.

[83] http://www.space-observer.de/ Was läuft falsch auf der Sone.26.07.2008

[84] http://www.klimaskeptiker.info/beitraege/labohm_skeptizismus.html

[85] http://wetterjournal.wordpress.com/2009/07/14/der-einfluss-des-im-mittel-208-jahrigen-de-vriessuess-zyklus-auf-das-klma-der-erde/

[86] Robinson A.B., Robinson N.E., and Soon,,,.: Environmental effects of increased atmospheric Carbon Dioxide, Journal of American Physicians and Surgeons, 12/2007, vol.12no3

[87] http://www.spiegel.de/wissenschaft/natur/0,1518,619630,00.html

[88] http://www.idruhr.de/nachrichten/detail/archive/2010/october/article/studie-sonnenzyklen-und-kosmische-strahlung-beeinflussen-den-klimawandel.html

[89] http://z-e-i-t-e-n-w-e-n-d-e.blogspot.com/2011/04/michio-kaku-massive-solar-flare-in.html

[90] http://www.waldportal.org/allgemein/news.allgemein2010/20100120/index

[91] http://www.waldportal.org/allgemein/news.allgemein2010/20100120/index

[92] http://www.waldportal.org/allgemein/news.allgemein2010/20100120/index

[93] http://www.g-o.de/inc/artikel_drucken.php?id=3506&a_flag=1

[94] http://www.derstandard.at/3140465/Urwald-Rodung-setzt-Milliarden-Tonnen-CO2-frei

[95] http://derstandard.at/3140465/Urwald-Rodung-setzt-Milliarden-Tonnen-CO2-frei

[96] Intergovernmental Panel on Climate Change (2007): IPCC Fourth Assessment Report – Working Group I Report "The Physical Science Basis"

[97] Hansen, J., Mki. Sato, R. Ruedy et al. (2005): Efficacy of climate forcings, in: Journal of Geophysical Research, 110, D18104, doi:10.1029/2005JD005776

[98] UNFCCC: Status of Ratification of the Kyoto Protocol

[99] Sueddeutsche Zeitung: Kanada steigt offiziell aus Kyoto Protokoll aus. 13.Dezember 2011

[100] http://www.ZeitenSchrift.com 51/06 Seite 32

[101] http://www.spiegel.de/wissenschaft/natur/0,1518,druck-619630,00.html.22.04.2009

[102] Bundesministerium für Umwelt, Naturschutz und Reaktorsicherheit. Mai 2011. IPCC – ein wissenschaftliches Gremium

[103] http://www.bmu.de/klimaschutz/internationale_klimapolitik/ipcc/doc/print/39274.php?

[104] http://www.sciencedaily.com/release/2012/05/120517111431.htm

[105] http://info.kopp-verlag.de/hintergruende/geostrategie/joanne-nova/die-auferstehung-des-ipcc-hckeystickbetrugs-in-australien.html.

[106] The Australian, Graham Lloyd, 17. September 2013

[107] John Edward Norwood Veron: A Reef in Time. The Great Barrier Reef from Beginning to End. Harvard University Press, Cambridge, Mass. 2008, ISBN

978-0-674-02679-7, p. 168.
[108] Zensur auf der Klimakonferenz: ZDF- und ARD-Chefredakteur protestieren bei Merkel und UNO. Gerhard Wisnewski. 18.12.2009
[109] http://www.leipzigerinstitut.de/wiki/daten/vorwort-freispruch-4.html
[110] http://nachrichten.t-online.de/friedensnobelpreis-fuer-barack-obama-aber-wofuer-genau-/id_20205674/index.09.10.2009
[111] http://nachrichten.t-online.de/friedensnobelpreis-fuer-barack-obama-aber-wofuer-genau-/id_20205674/index.09.10.2009
[112] APA-Copenhagen - Announcement dd. 13.03.2008

[113] http://www.science-explorer.de/reports/haarpprojekt.htm
[114] http://de.scribd.com/doc/57517637/Chemtrail-HAARP-Special
[115] http://de.scribd.com/doc/57517637/Chemtrail-HAARP-Special
[116] Deutscher Bundestag – 17. Wahlperiode Drucksache 17/10311 vom 16.07.2012
[117] Dr. Rosalie Bertell „Kriegswaffe Planet Erde" German Edition P. 323 12/2011
[118] Die neue Woche Nr.9 S15, 4.März 2014 Wissenschaft und Technik „Forscher: Manipulationen am Weltklima wenig effizient und gefährlich"
[119] Die neue Woche Nr.9 S15, 4.März 2014 Wissenschaft und Technik „Forscher: Manipulationen am Weltklima wenig effizient und gefährlich"